T0195096

What Causes Elevated Low Density Lipoproteins?

A Functional Nutrition Perspective

Gina Liberti, MS, AAS, MS ED

BALBOA.
PRESS

A DIVISION OF HAY HOUSE

Balboa Press books may be ordered through booksellers or by contacting:

Balboa Press
A Division of Hay House
1663 Liberty Drive
Bloomington, IN 47403
www.balboapress.com
1 (877) 407-4847

Print information available on the last page.

ISBN: 978-1-9822-3391-4 (sc)
ISBN: 978-1-9822-3392-1 (e)

Balboa Press rev. date: 08/27/2019

⊱⊱⊰

With the startling announcement in The New York Times[1], calling into question the value of some *'cholesterol'* lowering drugs, it would seem that nutrition professionals are in a unique and timely position; one that allows us to revisit the connection between diet, stress and lipoprotein levels. Artificially lowering lipoproteins does not explain why they are elevated in the first place. Pin pointing the role of food and nutrition in the development of this condition is therefore, essential, but perhaps, using a different perspective—a **Functional Nutrition** perspective. The Functional Nutrition model allows us to understand ***how the presence or absence of a substance in a food determines how the body uses that food.*** This model is a broad umbrella which includes the mathematics of energy potential, or the amount of calories provided by the number and sizes of servings. However, that potential is not emphasized. Instead, energy potential within the Functional Nutrition model is only a component of the overall picture—and hence, the Functional Nutrition model is a more biochemical model. For example, examine the difference between a refined and a whole grain. It is easy to see that the same amount of both grains contain within an almost equivalent energy potential. However, the whole grain, containing fiber, as well as an array of additional micronutrients, vitamins and minerals, will control how quickly the energy potential in the form of sugar enters the body, keeping blood sugar levels stable. Moreover, because of the micronutrients, the insulin will be used efficiently, creating a more effective and judicious way of producing energy, minimizing the potential to be stored as fat.

The Functional Nutrition model, as far as it influences our understanding of how food affects the body, also provides the means to determine how other factors are linked to the quality of nutritional choices. These factors include various forms of stress i.e. psychological, physical, oxidative, and toxic pollutants. Each additional influence and their associated biochemical products, places a greater load on the detoxification system. With increased detoxification needs, requirements for additional raw materials i.e. nutrients, also need to increase to support, not only detoxification, but *all* of the pathways that also rely on those nutrients. An easy way to visualize this is by looking at all biochemical pathways a *bills* that need to be *paid*. Nutrients represent the currency that pays those bills. Detoxification, because of its importance for maintaining the health of the body, could be considered the mortgage and all other bills would be of lesser value except for the stress response, which is a survival imperative. So if the detox bill is high, all available currency will be allocated to clear out the toxins, leaving no or very little resources to handle all the other bills i.e. regeneration of connected tissue, manufacture of red blood cells or even DNA synthesis.

Another example is the biochemical pathway methylation. This pathway is required to support phase 2 detoxification pathway. Within the liver, there is a two-step process for eliminating toxic substances from the body. Phase one prepares a fat loving or *lipophilic* toxin into something that is a more water soluble substance, referred to as a *biotransformed intermediate*. Phase two is involved in taking that biotransformed intermediate and further acting upon it through a processed referred to as conjugation. Utilizing *conjugases* or enzymes that facilitate the reaction, do so by attaching such molecules as sulfate, taurine, glutathione or *methyl groups*.[2],[3]

With Methylation, folate is a major substrate or a substance that works with enzymes to support biochemical reactions. But folate, indirectly in the active form, methyl folate, also acts as a cofactor, or a necessary ingredient in serotonin synthesis.[4],[5] With increased detoxification needs, requirements for folate also need to increase, or there may not be sufficient amounts to cover both detoxification reactions and serotonin synthesis. This may explain why low levels of folate have been linked to depression.[6],[7]

But how does the understanding of functionality relate to lipoproteins? We know that cholesterol is a component of both high (HDL) or low (LDL) density lipoprotein forms, along with *other* fat soluble products. The significance of this statement is that cholesterol is *not* LDL or HDL, since lipoproteins are compounds that function as lipid transport systems moving *all* fat soluble products in the blood. How each of these forms of lipoproteins function and how levels are altered by exercise or the presence or absence of certain nutrients becomes the focal point in understanding elevated levels of lipoproteins. The notion of good and bad becomes less important and instead, what influences appropriate levels of lipoproteins, from a nutrient excess or deficiency standpoint, becomes the issue. With this in mind, along with the new revelations that some lipoprotein lowering drugs may not be able to decrease mortality[8], it seems prudent to explore how nutrient deficiencies or excesses or the need for more raw materials contribute to a change in lipoprotein levels in the body.

The purpose of cholesterol

It is well understood that cholesterol is an important component of our bodies performing such tasks as providing the raw materials for adrenal and sex hormones and vitamin D. [9],[10] Cholesterol is used to form myelin sheaths[11] and without bile, which also includes cholesterol as an ingredient, we would be unable to digest dietary fat or absorb fat soluble vitamins. [12] Cholesterol functions in stabilizing cell membranes [13] compensating for changes in the fluidity of the membranes. In fact, this function is so important that, while the liver is the main site of synthesis with contributions of approximately 80%, [14] nearly every cell membrane has the ability to synthesize cholesterol.[15] And, as dietary cholesterol *decreases*, the negative feedback will stimulate the activity of the enzyme, HMG Co A reductase (3-hydroxy-3-methylglutaryl-CoA reductase), to *increase* its synthesis by the liver. [16]

In the skin, cholesterol not only water proofs our cells, [17],[18] protecting us from the elements as well as dehydration, it also assists in the healing of skin tissue while preventing infection from harmful microorganisms. [19]

Studies done at Baylor College of Medicine have revealed the critical role of cholesterol in the developing infant's brain and myelin sheaths around nerves. Interestingly, this research also showed that typically increased levels of cholesterol in mother's milk caused elevated LDL levels but *not* HDL levels. In the infant, it seems that they use cholesterol differently than adults and because of its importance in early development there seems to be a down-regulating mechanism with an increased dietary load. These data gives rise to questions about the potential for lipoprotein problems later in life, if low cholesterol formula is used instead of mother's milk, causing the infant to compensate by producing more. Cholesterol rich mother's milk may actually provide protection in later life.[20]

Additionally, a decrease in membrane cholesterol levels appears to be associated with a decrease in the number of serotonin receptors, indicating a possible link between low levels of cholesterol, depression and suicide. [21], [22] Several recent studies have focused on the role of cholesterol in proper signaling complexes, revealing a critical role in cellular communication. [23],[24],[25] This role may illustrate how cholesterol assists in preventing cancer, since a breakdown in cellular communication is part of a sequence of events that appears to influence the development of a cancerous cell. [26],[27] In fact, newer research has indicated that artificial lowering of Low Density Lipoprotein levels with statin drugs, may increase the risk of cancer. [28],[29]

Elevated levels of low density lipoproteins are often seen during times of prolonged stress. A recent study has identified that cholesterol may play a protective role with the immune system. Cholesterol appears to be an important factor in cross-presentation: an activity that increases the activation of T cells. [30] Since chronic stress can impair the immune system, it would seem that a connection between high levels of cholesterol during times of stress could be a protective measure against viruses or mutations.[31],[32], [33] This may be particularly significant with vitamin D levels since recent research suggests that this vitamin has anti-viral activity.[34]

And lastly, cholesterol is susceptible to oxidation when vitamin and mineral status is low (i.e., vitamin C, vitamin E, selenium, zinc).[35] Since antioxidants are critical for protecting against oxidative damage linked to the development of heart disease[36] and cancer[37], this activity may not only explain why lipoprotein levels increase as we age, but may also illustrate a link between lower levels and increased oxidative stress as a result of low serum antioxidant reserves.

With all of these important roles in mind, perhaps it would be prudent to view Low Density Lipoproteins as the equivalent of a *UPS* truck making deliveries to various sites to be used as a raw material for structural components, hormones and other regulatory substances. High density lipoproteins are the equivalent of *Fed Ex* vans picking up the unused left over cholesterol that is no longer needed to be disposed of. That means that elevated levels of low density lipoproteins are *not a disease, but, instead a marker for some kind of imbalance in the body or an increased need for raw materials.*

The Role of Inflammation in the development of Elevated Lipoproteins

Inflammation is an intricate biochemical and cellular response to a variety of injury-causing stimuli,[38] and can only occur in vascularized and perfused tissue.[39] It is a process designed to remove the cause of the reaction while inducing a healing response. Although an appropriate response (as opposed to an exaggerated inflammatory reaction) is capable of initiating tissue regeneration or repair, it can still cause pain and endanger healthy tissue.[40] In general, chronic inflammation differs from acute by the amount of time each type persists, with a chronic response lasting for at least two weeks.[41] The causes of inflammation range from various immunological reactions, chemical agents, and toxins, to mechanical trauma, heat, X-rays and ultraviolet light. Whatever the cause, once inflammation occurs, plasma proteins (C-reactive protein) and leukocytes (white blood cells), along with their biochemical mediators appear.[42] These biochemical mediators include cytokines, a class of proteins that are involved in communication activities among macrophages, as well as different subsets of lymphocytes. As part of the immune response, cytokines (interleukins, tumor necrosis factor and interferon), bind with specific receptors on target cells providing genetically programmed instructions to these cells on how to behave.[43]

Current research has indicated that there is a link between inflammation and elevated levels of Low Density Lipoproteins (LDL).[44] In fact, when an inflammatory response develops, a number of changes in lipid and lipoprotein activity also occur. For example: cytokines, through the release of the enzyme HMG Co A reductase, stimulate an increase in the synthesis of hepatic cholesterol, while simultaneously preventing the activity of cholesterol 7 alpha-hydroxylase, an important enzyme involved in the synthesis of bile. Hepatic lipase activity decreases, and not only do High Density Lipoprotein (HDL) levels decrease, but their metabolism is altered, as well.[45] Also, the levels of apolipoprotein A1, a major constituent of HDLs in plasma levels, appear to decrease. This is significant since apolipoprotein A1 is a cofactor for lecithin-cholesterol acyltransferase (LCAT)[46], a transport system by which free cholesterol is *esterfied* so it can be more readily returned to the liver. Another alteration in HDL function involves serum amyloid A (SAA), a type of HDL apolipoprotein.[47] This class of acute phase proteins can sharply escalate in the blood in response to inflammation,[48] and can participate in such activities as transporting cholesterol to the liver to be used in the synthesis of bile.[49] In the presence of inflammation and/or infection, these SAA proteins are also capable of behaving like a cytokine influencing a variety of activities that contribute to the development of atherosclerosis.[50,51]

Interestingly, these changes in lipids and lipoprotein metabolism may provide some benefits. There are some studies that suggest that the increase in the biosynthesis of cholesterol may offer protection from the adverse effects of various pathogenic organisms,[52],[53] and be associated with tissue repair, [54],[55] particularly in the presence of metabolic syndrome.[56]

What is important here is that this information suggests that *anything* that chronically initiates an inflammatory state could be associated with the development of elevated low density lipoproteins or LDLs.

Immune Response

As previously stated, inflammation can occur from a variety of circumstances ranging from physical injury to intense heat, toxins and heavy metal exposure or an **immune challenge**. [57] In fact, inflammation is considered a hallmark of an immune response, indicating that an infection, allergy or sensitivity to a food or other substances can initiate an inflammatory state in the body. Given the relationship between inflammation and cholesterol, it would be prudent to explore the role of an immune challenge with the development of elevated lipoproteins. Regarding food, an immune response can be a classical allergy (immediate response IgE mediated) or a sensitivity (delayed IgG mediated). [58] With a classical allergy or immediate, IgE response, such symptoms as swelling, rashes or anaphylaxis can be observed. With a delayed IgG response, vague symptoms can be observed hours, or days after the food in question is ingested.[59] The significance of a delayed IgG mediated response is two-fold: first, if a response is delayed, then it may be more difficult to pinpoint a certain food(s) as the instigator of an inflammatory response. Second, IgG mediated responses are associated with activating the *complement cascade*, or an activated sequence that enhances the inflammatory response.[60] This information suggests that chronic inflammation from an *unrecognized* food sensitivity, could indirectly effect LDL levels.

There is a great deal of current research pinpointing the relationship between bacterial endotoxins and hyperlipidemia. The term endotoxin can refer to the lipopolysaccharide (LPS) portion of the outer membrane or structural component of gram negative bacteria such as *Shigella, Salmonella,* and *E. coli*. But in general, endotoxin is used to describe any cell-associated bacterial toxin that is liberated after the bacteria is lysed. [61], [62] When present, they initiate the activity of a number of proteins: Toll-like receptor 4 (TLR-4) and LPS binding protein (LBP). TLR-4 and LBP are capable of initiating signaling pathways that involve protein kinases, which ultimately activate nuclear factor kappa-B (NFK-B)[63]. Kinases are a class of enzymes involved in the regulation of cellular pathways involving cellular communication,[64] and NFK-B is a transcription factor, or protein, that regulates the expression of inflammatory mediators.[65] With multiple sources of instigating and maintaining inflammation in the body, it is possible that there are many ways that increased need for cholesterol and transport during an immune response can occur.

Oxidative Stress

Oxidative stress is a term used to describe an over abundance of free radicals and not enough antioxidants to protect the body from the effects of their instability [66]. There is a wealth of research linking oxidative stress and elevated LDLs. [67], [68], [69] In fact, according to the cardiologist, Dr. Stephen Sinatra in his book, ***Lower Your Blood Pressure in Eight Weeks***: "We now realize that LDL cholesterol isn't dangerous in its own right. It's only when LDL cholesterol becomes oxidized that it becomes a danger to your circulatory system." [70] He further explains that oxidized LDL cholesterol (LDL-C) is so irritating to the lining of blood vessels, the resultant inflammation leads to the development of fatty streaks—the forerunner of atherosclerosis. But this explanation is only part of the picture, since oxidized LDL can have an effect on HDL metabolism, interfering with the reverse cholesterol transport system. In this system, as previously described, the aforementioned LCAT enzyme modulates the conversion of free cholesterol, to the more readily accepted esterified form. Esterified cholesterol, via HDL particles are then transported to the liver. Inhibition of this enzyme due to oxidation is associated with the accumulation of free cholesterol which is strongly linked with the development of atherosclerosis. [71], [72] Additionally, oxidation can also affect the activity of lipoprotein A-1, which acts as a cofactor, or a necessary component for initiating enzymes, in the activity of LCAT. The affect of oxidation on the activity of this substance is believed to occur through the formation of crosslinks or a process by which tissues are irreversibly damaged. [73], [74] In either case, the reverse cholesterol transport system is impaired effecting cholesterol clearance.

Stress

As previously mentioned, **increased stress levels** are also associated with the development of hyperlipidemia. [75] In an acute stress situation lipoproteins can sharply elevate, as recounted in a 2005 article written for *The Journal of Alternative and Complementary Medicine*, by Annemarie Colbin, PhD. Here, Dr. Colbin had interviewed the previously mentioned Dr. Stephen Sinatra. He described that while performing a stressful 6 hour cardiac surgery, he had discovered that his LDL levels rose from 180mg/dl to 240 mg/dl, even though he had not eaten any food.[76]

There also appears to be a connection between chronic *psychological stress* and chronic inflammation. [77] Although intermittent stress is a component of survival, it is not the same thing as prolonged stress associated with modern living. [78] In fact, current research has been focusing on the notion of *allostasis*, or being able to create stability through change, as a result of both acute and chronic alterations in the stress response system.[79] The stress response reflects an active and dynamic interaction between a wide range of systems. These systems include the hypothalamic-pituitary-adrenal axes or HPA axis and the cardiovascular, metabolic, autonomic and immune systems. [80], [81], [82] The idea is that if the immune system, autonomic nervous system and the HPA axis, are all chronically *dysregulated,* then chronic *alterations* in metabolism and levels of inflammation can occur. This multi-system dysregulation then interacts with other influences like diet and genetics; creating the environment for a variety of diseases to develop, in particular metabolic syndrome.[83]

Also known as Syndrome X, metabolic syndrome refers to a clustering of symptoms that include insulin resistance, hyperlipidemia, obesity, abnormalities in clotting which may or may not be associated with hypertension, all in the *absence* of diabetes.[84] With chronic stress, there is an increase in the level of glucocorticoids, or a class of steroid hormones, which tends to increase the storage of fats in the visceral, or abdominal area rather than subcutaneous adipose tissue. [85] And it is visceral fat that expresses higher levels of Tumor Necrosis Factor-alpha (TNF-alpha), which is directly related to inflammation[86], cardiovascular disease and elevated levels of lipoproteins. [87], [88]

Blood pH Levels

Somewhat controversial is the idea that the inflammatory state can be associated with **low pH levels in the blood**. And while there is no direct evidence to support this notion, there is research that indicates that there is such a thing as chronic low–level metabolic acidosis,[89] and that such conditions are associated with diets that provide insufficient amounts of fruits and vegetables with an emphasis on refined starches and proteins.[90, 91, 92] This type of diet has also been linked with the development of insulin resistance,[93] a condition commonly associated with elevated levels of lipoproteins. [94, 95] There is also research that shows a connection between acidosis and hypothyroidism, which may suggest a link between chronic low pH levels and thyroid function. And while acidosis is generally thought of as a severe metabolic imbalance, this condition does offer insight into the relationship between blood pH and physiological function. It seems clear that there is a need for more research linking the role of sub-clinical acidosis to both the presence of inflammation and hypothyroidism. Particularly since low thyroid function is also associated with hyperlipidemia. [96, 97]

Increased consumption of sugar and refined carbohydrates

It seems certain that sugar has the capacity to participate in a chain of events that causes an inflammatory state, such as increasing cortisol, the catecholamines epinephrine and norepinephrine, as well as inflammatory markers like TNF-alpha, and interleukin-6 (IL-6). Chronic ingestion of sugar and refined carbohydrates have also been associated with the elevation of coagulation substances such as fibrinogen and an inhibitor of fibrinolysis, plasminogen activator inhibitor – 1 (PAI-1) [98], both of which have been associated with hyperlipidemia. [99, 100] Regardeing cortisol: while it is a steroid which is anti inflammatory, there has been some very compelling research looking at chronic cortisol and the upregulation of T Helper type 2 (Th2) cells associated with inflammation.[101]

Interestingly, where there appears to be a lack of direct evidence with sugar, the reverse has been demonstrated: diets that are high in fiber, which acts as a controlling mechanism for how quickly sugar enters the body, and low glycemic index carbohydrates, both appear to reduce the presence of inflammation. [102], [103], [104]

But, the research linking fructose to inflammation appears to be much clearer, indicating that by itself, in conjunction with refined carbohydrates or *magnesium* deficiency, dietary fructose can increase inflammation. [105], [106], [107], [108] Additionally, while fructose does not stimulate the secretion of insulin, the concomitant release of leptin is inhibited, preventing the regulatory signal that curbs appetite. [109] Moreover, recent research has shown that fructose in amounts of at least 50% of the diet can increase PPARγ co-activator 1α and 1β (PGC-1α and PGC-1β) which not only causes lipogenesis but insulin resistance, as well.[110] PPAR or peroxisome proliferator-activated receptors are a group of receptors that respond to various hormones ultimately stimulating genetic expression. PPARγ, in particular is involved in adipose tissue production and an increase in the storage of fat.[111]

Considering this, however, it is also important to note that fructose as a common monosaccharide of many foods, most notably fruits and vegetables, is not the same thing as fructose isolated from corn and added as an inexpensive sweetener to manufactured foods. In fact, the form of fructose commonly used, particularly in soft drinks and processed desserts, is high fructose corn sweetener (HFCS). This form of fructose is not a pure product, but is instead, a combination of glucose, fructose and various oligosaccharides. [112] This form of fructose often accounts for a total dietary intake of about 20% [113] and greater than 50% of sweetener intake, linking its use to the increase in the prevalence of obesity and insulin resistance. [114] While this form of sweetener has declined sharply in the last 10 years, it is still used in a variety of products including sodas, some salad dressings and condiments, bread and other wheat products, nut butters and prepackaged goods. [115]

In general, however, excessive amounts of sugar and refined carbohydrates have been associated with the development of obesity, particularly in the absence of physical activity. [116] So while there may be no direct link between sugar and refined carbohydrates and lipoprotein levels, there are indirect links that bear consideration.

Obesity

Adipose tissue has long been considered an inert substance, acting as insulation, as well as involved in the storage of energy. But researchers have now come to understand that it is, in fact, an endocrine organ, capable of synthesizing and secreting a number of hormones, and that these hormones can have an influence on our moods[117], appetite, reproductive functions, immune response, and energy levels.[118],[119] In particular, the adipokine secretion of pro-inflammatory IL-6 is linked to insulin resistance. [120] In fact, the presence of IL-6 along with TNF-alpha, appear to be able to foretell the future progression of not just obesity, but diabetes, as well. [121] The mechanism of this appears to be associated with TNF-alpha interfering with the proper function of insulin receptor, various insulin receptor substrates, as well as sustained activation of stress related kinases, that are pro-inflammatory in nature.[122] Adipokines are a class of compounds that regulate lipoprotein metabolism, and are secreted by adipocytes, or cells that store fat. [123]

Research has not only shown that the loss of weight can reduce inflammatory markers,[124], [125], [126] but that other parameters are also improved. Weight loss can increase insulin sensitivity [127] as well as levels of the protein adiponectin—a substance only secreted by adipocytes, capable of regulating glucose and lipid metabolism. [128] It is involved in insulin responsiveness as well as reducing the production of cellular inflammation within blood vessels. [129], [130] However, there is compelling research that suggests that this benefit may not extend to elderly men, [131] indicating that adiponectin may not necessarily confer benefits to everyone. But what is clear, is that weight loss has also been shown to improve lipid profile. [132], [133]

Finally, the consumption of fructose needs to be revisited as a means for increasing the prevalence of obesity. It is well known by nutrition professionals that fructose is not metabolized the same way as glucose. In fact, it not only does not require insulin for metabolism, but the liver is the only organ that can metabolize it. While this has been considered beneficial in the short term, particularly for diabetics, it does not seem to be the case with chronic ingestion. Under the control of phosphofructokinase, gluco-6-phosphate is converted to fructose -1-6- bisphosphate, making it possible for fructose to continuously enter the glycolytic pathway.[134],[135] From there, de novo lipogenesis occurs increasing the production of Very Low Density Lipoproteins (the precursor to low density lipoproteins).[136], [137] Additionally, it has been a common practice to use sugar alcohols such as sorbitol and mannitol in place of sugar because they have less calories per gram than fructose or sucrose. However, these alternative sweeteners are easily converted to fructose by the liver. [138]

Insulin Resistance

As previously stated, obesity can lead to insulin resistance or a reduced capacity for recognizing and allowing the transport of glucose from the blood into the cells to be used for fuel. [139] But an important question to ask is: what came first, obesity leading to insulin resistance or insulin resistance leading to the development of obesity. Or could there be some other underlying cause? These questions are significant because there are a number of studies indicating that insulin resistance can occur with individuals who are *not* obese, indicating that there may be the presence of something else that can lead to the development of insulin resistance and that something else appears to be a chronic *subclinical* inflammatory state. [140],[141] Various health conditions, such as psoriasis, pre-hypertension and non-alcoholic fatty liver have been associated with insulin resistance, in the *absence* of obesity, with C-reactive protein as a common inflammatory marker. [142],[143],[144].

Another aspect of the development of insulin resistance is something that is well understood by nutrition professionals; that the development of this condition, in some circumstances, can be related to chromium status.[145] In fact, studies have shown that compared to those *without* type 2 diabetes, those with insulin resistance, tend to have lower blood levels of chromium.[146] There also is evidence to suggest that chromium status decreases as we age,[147] and considering the fact that chromium requires stomach acid for proper absorption, it is no surprise that age can be a factor in the status of this mineral, since it is not uncommon for hydrochloric acid levels to decrease with age.[148] In addition, enhanced urinary excretion of chromium is associated with increased levels of circulating sugar and insulin.[149]

There are multiple studies that indicate that chromium enhances insulin responsiveness but the mechanism appears to be unclear. It seems that a cascade of events occurs, starting with the transport of chromium via transferrin to cell membranes, where it binds to low-molecular-weight chromium-binding substance (LMWCr) creating its apo or inactive form.[150],[151] Once bound to the LMWCr oligopeptide, chromodulin (the active form) is synthesized, and its binding to insulin activated insulin receptors causes the activation of tyrosine kinase. With activation of tyrosine kinase, insulin receptor substrate-1 is phosphorylated, increasing the activity of glucose transport 4 (GLUT 4) molecules, raising the uptake of glucose from the blood into the membranes of such insulin responsive tissues as adipose and muscle cells.[152] Chromium has also been shown to inhibit the enzyme phosphotyrosine phosphatase, which has been linked to decrease insulin sensitivity. [153]

Vitamin E deficiency

It is commonly believed that vitamin E deficiency is rare due to its wide spread presence in a variety of foods. But there is some indication that this notion may not be entirely true. First of all, recommendations for increasing the amounts of polyunsaturated fats have grown significantly, and with the increase in these fatty acids, there needs to be an increase in vitamin E to protect against peroxidation.[154] Low fat diets also limit the amount of vitamin E, as well as losses due to refinement of whole grains, which can range from 35 - 90 %[155], or more. [156] Exposure to air, prolonged heat and freezing can also compromise vitamin E levels in foods.[157]

Besides being an important protector against oxidation of LDLs, vitamin E also participates in other activities that help to prevent inflammation. There is evidence to suggest that vitamin E is capable of influencing such enzymes as cyclooxygenase 2 (COX-2) and 5-Lipooxygenase (5-LO), both associated with the production of inflammation. [158] And *gamma* tocopherol, in particular, has demonstrated inhibition of TNF-alpha and Prostaglandin E2 (PGE2) and appears to reduce inflammation-mediated damage in rats.[159] While gamma tocopherol represents 70% of the form of vitamin E found in food[160], the form of vitamin E commonly used in nutritional supplements is *alpha* tocopherol, a form that when given alone, has been found to deplete gamma tocopherol in the body.[161]

Gina Liberti, MS, AAS, MS ED

Vitamin D Deficiency

Although vitamin D is best known for its association with calcium utilization and bone density, more recent research is showing a link between vitamin D status and insulin utilization, [162], [163] as well as other health conditions such as hyperparathyroidism [164], gestational diabetes [165], and pre-eclampsia[166], [167]. Regarding insulin activity, vitamin D deficiency has been shown to blunt insulin synthesis, and particularly in early life, such deficiencies have been associated with the development of type 1 diabetes, later on[168]. Additionally, serum 25-hydroxyvitamin D (25-OHD) levels have been shown to be inversely related to a variety of such parameters leading to the development of diabetes as body mass index (BMI), body fat content, and insulin resistance,[169] all of which are associated with inflammation.

Of great concern is the growing awareness that vitamin D deficiency is widespread. According the Michael Holick, MD, PhD, of Boston University School of Medicine, vitamin D deficiency is epidemic in America. [170] He suggests that "…judicious limited exposure to sunlight as the best method to prevent vitamin D deficiency. Since the cutaneous production of vitamin D3 is dependent on so many factors, including season, time of day, latitude, and the person's sensitivity to sunlight (i.e. pigmentation), no one recommendation can be made. If a person knows that he/she will develop a mild sunburn minimum erythemal dose (MED) after 30 minutes of sun exposure, then exposure of the face, arms, hands, and legs for 20% to 25% of that time (i.e. 6 to 8 minutes) 2 to 3 times a week is more than adequate to satisfy the body's requirement. A sunscreen with a sun protection factor of 15 can then be applied to prevent the damaging effects of excessive sun exposure." [171]

Those that are at risk for developing a vitamin D deficiency include the elderly who may not be able to efficiently produce the vitamin in the presence of UVB radiation. Dark skinned individuals, excessive use of sun screen, location and time of year as well as the presence of inflammatory bowel disease can also effect vitamin D status.[172],[173] Vitamin D is, therefore, conditionally essential as a nutrient.

Results in the field of cancer research, however, has indicated two significant facts regarding vitamin D. First, it appears that vitamin D has antioxidant activity. [174] And second, that endogenous vitamin D production can be upregulated by increasing the amount of isoflavones in the diet. In fact, both genistein and resveratrol have been shown to exert influence over 2 different enzymes CYP24 and CYP27B1, both of which belong to the cytochrome p450 enzyme family. This family of enzymes are associated with most phase one detoxification reactions.[175] The former enzyme, CYP24, involved in the degradation of 1, 25-dihydroxyvitamin D3, as well as its precursor, 25- (OH) -D3, to an inactive aggregate, is inhibited. And the latter CYP27B1 enzyme, which is involved in the synthesis of 1, 25-dihydroxyvitamin D3, is upregulated, suggesting that its increased activity may also stimulate an increase in the synthesis of this most active form of vitamin D, as well. [176]

Because there is concern that too much supplemental vitamin D has been linked to an increase in the deposition of calcium into the soft tissue of the kidneys, heart, blood vessels, and the lung,[177] upper limits have been set for various age groups. This concern may be unwarranted since more scrutiny of the role of vitamin K2, menaquinone, has suggested that its status in the body is associated with reduced vascular calcification. And while this research is in its infancy, it is showing promise.[178] However, there is some controversy over the change in recommended upper levels from 2011 to the current recommended levels. [179]

Below compares the two different recommendations:

2011:

- 0-6 months – 1000 IU
- 7-12 months -1,500 IU
- 1-3 years – 2,500 IU
- 4-8 years – 3,000 IU
- 9 or > - 4,000 IU [180]

Current Adequate intakes (AI):[181]

Table 2: Recommended Dietary Allowances (RDAs) for Vitamin D

Age	Male	Female	Pregnancy	Lactation
0–12 months*	400 IU (10 mcg)	400 IU (10 mcg)		
1–13 years	600 IU (15 mcg)	600 IU (15 mcg)		
14–18 years	600 IU (15 mcg)	600 IU (15 mcg)	600 IU (15 mcg)	600 IU (15 mcg)
19–50 years	600 IU (15 mcg)	600 IU (15 mcg)	600 IU (15 mcg)	600 IU (15 mcg)
51–70 years	600 IU (15 mcg)	600 IU (15 mcg)		
>70 years	800 IU (20 mcg)	800 IU (20 mcg)		

Insomnia

Studies have shown that sleep deprivation is associated with a disturbance in endocrine function that leads to increased

Inflammation. Plasma levels of leptin (a hormone associated with the regulation of appetite in relation to the amount of fat in the body)[182] tend to decrease while levels of ghrelin (a gastric hormone that stimulates the secretion of pituitary growth hormone that increases hunger and food intake)[183] have been shown to increase. An increase in appetite appears to further complicate the situation since sleep deprivation is also associated with impaired carbohydrate tolerance. [184], [185] Additionally, after a night of sleep loss, monocyte production of TNF-alpha and the pro-inflammatory cytokine, IL-6 have both been shown to be elevated, as compared to blood levels after a night of uninterrupted sleep.[186]

Magnesium deficiency

Magnesium is a critical cofactor in multiple biochemical reactions from energy production and detoxification reactions to the synthesis of protein and DNA. But more recent research has shown a direct correlation between low levels of magnesium and the development of inflammation. Studies have shown that a deficiency in this mineral initiates what has been termed a *clinical inflammatory syndrome* which has been characterized as the activation of polymorphonuclear leukocytes and macrophages.[187] The presence of macrophages initiates acute phase proteins, like interleukins, TNF-alpha, and inflammatory cytokines. [188], [189] Where upon the liver responds by producing a number of acute phase reactants, such as coagulation and complement factors and C-reactive protein. [190] This inflammatory response also appears to initiate a reduction in plasma antioxidants[191], most notably super oxide dismutase and reduced glutathione. [192]

Magnesium status is also associated with insulin activity, acting as a cofactor in the cell membrane glucose transport system as well as participating in reactions that involve carbohydrate oxidation. Not only does insulin secretion, binding and activity depend on magnesium,[193] but conversely, magnesium requires insulin for its uptake into tissues that are insulin sensitive. [194] In fact, poor intracellular magnesium levels are commonly found with non insulin dependent diabetes. The mechanism appears to be associated with both defective tyrosine-kinase activity, as well as increased intracellular calcium concentrations. And there is evidence to suggest that magnesium may act as a natural calcium channel blocker. [195,196] These two conditions appear to be responsible for defective insulin activity and the exacerbation of insulin resistance. [197]

There is some evidence to suggest that magnesium status may also be associated with insomnia and that the connection is with either hypo or hyperfunction of the biological clock. [198] Additionally, magnesium status may also be compromised by low blood pH. There is evidence to suggest that the acid-base status can effect magnesium excretion without regard to the intake of this mineral, and that the elderly, in particular, may be at increased risk for a deficiency. [199]

Omega-3 and omega-6 fatty acid imbalance

Omega 3 and 6 fatty acids cannot be manufactured by the body and must be supplied in the diet. The ratio between these two types of essential fatty acids have been listed anywhere between (depending on the source) 1:1 and 5:1[200], with the omega-3 being the smaller or of equal value to the omega-6. The discrepancy appears to be due to the fact that different areas within the body have different requirements. For example, the ratio of omega 6 to omega 3 in adipose tissue is 5:1 and within the brain, 1:1.[201] However, since the delta 6 desaturase enzyme converts omega 3 fatty acids to eicosapentaenoic acid (EPA) and docosahexanoic acid (DHA) four times as quickly as omega 6 fatty acids are converted to gamma-linolenic acid, ideally the ratio should be 4:1 in our foods in order to achieve equal conversion. [202] However, the typical American diet boasts of a ratio anywhere between 10:1 and 25:1 or even as high as 30:1, (with the omega-6 being the fatty acid in excess) creating a pro-inflammatory state. [203],[204] Although this is gradually changing, the imbalance has been thought to be due primarily to the increased presence of grain fed animals in our food supply[205],[206] and an increase in the use of vegetable seed oils, soybean and corn products. [207]

It has been known for some time that the active form of omega 3 fatty acid, eicosapentaenoic acid (EPA) is capable of decreasing the production of prostaglandin E2 (PGE2), by inhibiting the release of arachidonic acid from membranes. Its release and subsequent production of PGE2 is a potent instigator of inflammation. [208]

However, there is other anti inflammatory activity associated with omega 3 fatty acid that is not completely clear. There appears to be a relationship between this fatty acid and inhibition in the rise of TNF-alpha gene expression, as well as an increase in adiponectin levels. This activity may be due to the activation of peroxisome proliferator-activated receptor alpha (PPAR-alpha)[209], which has been shown to reduce insulin resistance[210]. This may further explain the link between magnesium and insulin resistance since *phytol*, a component of chlorophyll, upregulates PPAR-alpha.[211] Other recent research has shown that in addition to lowering TNF-alpha, other inflammatory markers, IL-1 beta and IL-6, were also inhibited by alpha linolenic acid.[212] And omega 3 fatty acids have been shown to improve impaired glucose tolerance. [213],[214]

Another consideration is the ability of the body to take alpha linolenic acid (ALA) and convert it to its active form EPA and DHA. The body requires the minerals magnesium and zinc and the vitamins B3, B6 and vitamin C for the conversion to occur. If there are insufficient raw materials available, a functional deficiency can exist even though there may be ample amounts of omega 3 fatty acid in the diet.[215] Of additional concern is the growing trend to significantly reduce omega 3 fatty acids from food due to its high susceptibility to oxidation. The removal has been done through the genetic modification of both soy and canola beans. Iowa State University has dedicated 30 years of research in the development of a low linolenic acid soy bean reducing the normal 7-8% of ALA to only 1%. [216,217] Kellogg's has been using the low *lin* soybean oil since 2005 [218] and Kentucky Fried Chicken has been using it since 2006.[219] A canola variety called high oleic canola oil, has been developed with reduced alpha linoleic and linolenic acids and an increase in oleic acid.[220] So while both soybean and canola oils are recommended for their heart healthy omega 3 fatty acid content, they may not necessarily provide the protection they are thought to offer, because the ALA content has been reduced. [221]

Insufficient Amounts of Phytosterols

Phytosterols are a type of lipid that are naturally occurring in plants. They are part of the same family of compounds referred to as steroids, which also includes cholesterol. [222] While there have been more than 40 phytosterols identified, the most abundant and effective of this class of compounds for reducing low density lipoprotein levels are *B*-sitosterol, campesterol and stigmasterol.[223] Sterols work by displacing cholesterol from micelles and as a result, intestinal cholesterol absorption is reduced and fecal cholesterol excretion is increased. [224]

Stanols, a naturally occurring hydrogenated form of sterols, are much less abundant in nature, but have also shown the ability to lower low density lipoproteins. [225] While both sterols and stanols occur in the same foods: fruits, vegetables, nuts and seeds, vegetable oils, legumes and whole grains, there is a question as to the ability to derive sufficient amounts by consuming a variety of whole plants foods. In order to obtain 100 mg of plant sterols, it is necessary to consume 200 grams of additive free flours and between 500 and 700 grams or about a pound to a pound and a half of fresh fruits and vegetables. [226]

There has also been evidence that phytosterols have the ability to modulate immune function, which includes inhibiting the inflammatory response. [227] In nature, sterols exist in combination with beta-sisterolin (sterolins), which is a glucoside. The relationship between sterols and glucosides (any sugar bound to another compound) is what allows phytosterols to have their beneficial effect on the immune system; including the modulation of cortisol, and its concurrent effects on interleukin-6, an inflammatory cytokine. [228]

While there is little information about the effect of cooking and storage on the levels of phytosterols in food, there is some evidence that suggests that these compounds may be sensitive to boiling, where they can be lost in the cooking water. There are also concerns that food processing, in general, and the freezing of vegetables and fruits, in particular can cause the destruction of the glucoside molecules and their immuno-modulating activity. [229]

Gina Liberti, MS, AAS, MS ED

A Diet High in Trans Fatty Acids

Studies in the 1990s illustrated a connection between the use of artificially hydrogenated oils and lipoprotein levels in the body. [230],[231],[232] In fact, there has been ample research indicating that trans fatty acids not only raise LDL levels, lower HDL levels, [233] but also adversely effect the LDL:HDL ratio, [234] making these artificial fats highly atherogenic. These alterations appear to be associated with increased catabolism of Apolipoprotein A-1. In addition, there is a decrease in the catabolism of Apolipoprotein B-100, a major constituent of LDL involved in the solubilization of cholesterol within the LDL complex facilitating the subsequent deposition on the arterial wall. [235] There is also evidence to suggest that trans fatty acids not only increase the accumulation of cholesterol within the cell, but the secretion of free cholesterol and cholesterol esters by liver cells, as well. [236]

Clearly, there appears to be a variety of mechanisms at play and while they are generally not well understood, it is known that trans fatty acids can inhibit the delta 6 desaturase enzyme, responsible for converting omega 3 and 6 fatty acids to their elongated or active forms. This inhibition, thus contributes to the deleterious effects of essential fatty acid deficiency. [237] Regarding an increase of triglycerides and VLDL molecules, a partial explanation in their upregulation appears to be an association with the elevation of mRNA of fatty acid synthase, which catalyzes the last step in fatty acid synthesis and microsomal transfer protein mRNA, involved in the regulation of very low density lipoprotein assembly in the liver. [238]

While it appears that researchers recognize the connection between trans fats and insulin resistance, results from available studies have been inconsistent. [239] However, one study does appear to indicate two possible mechanisms involved with this connection. First, there is evidence suggesting a reduction in both the cardiac content of glucose transporter -4, the most significant transporter of insulin-regulated glucose[240], and in the hepatic content of glycogen. [241] This is important because glycogen is used for energy during unpredictable strenuous activity and is readily available for that purpose. [242]

And finally, of all of the varied information associated with the harmful effects of trans fatty acids and lipoprotein levels, there seems to be some agreement regarding the elevation of inflammatory markers. Such markers are C-reactive protein (CRP), TNF alpha receptors 1 and 2, IL-6, and IL-1 receptor agonist.[243] Additionally, there also appears to be an increase of monocyte chemoattractant protein 1, a cytokine that through the production of inflammatory chemicals attracts white blood cells to the site of an injury. There is also an increase in brain naturietic peptide (BNP), a cardiac neuron-hormone that is released by the cardiac myocytes due to an increase in ventricle volume pressure overload, and a concomitant increase in wall tension.[244] It functions to assist in keeping blood vessels dilated. Of note, is that BNP appears to be expressed in the presence of Prostaglandin E2, a hormone-like substance that is released in the presence of inflammation. [245]

Deficiency of B vitamins

In 1969, Dr. Kilmer McCully published an article, discussing the connection between certain B vitamin deficiencies and elevated levels of homocysteine, a bi-product of methionine metabolism. In that article, Dr. McCully suggested that elevated levels of homocysteine was a much more significant risk factor for the development of atherosclerosis than fat and cholesterol. Needless to say, the theory was not well accepted. Over thirty years later, numerous studies have supported Dr. McCully's research.[246]

The effect of hyperhomocysteinemia on lipotprotein activity begins with the increase in inflammation. It is related to the production of the derivative, *homocysteine thiolactone*, which is associated with elevated levels of oxidation. Through a number of inhibitory actions, thiolactone induced oxidation has been associated with the injury of a critical regulator of insulin activity: insulin-stimulated phosphatidylinositol 3-kinase, leading to insulin resistance.[247] In addition, the production of thiolactone has also been shown to interfere with the biosynthesis of protein, and the ensuing damage induces an immune response.[248] Apoptosis, or programmed cell death, is also a part of this equation, particularly since oxidative stress can induce programmed cell death. [249],[250] Additionally, homocysteine thiolactone is excreted through urine, [251] and high levels in the blood can be associated with kidney disease.[252]

But homocysteine levels are also associated with hepatic steatosis, [253], [254] or an abnormal synthesis and breakdown of fat causing increased lipid retention within the liver.[255] The mechanism involved is associated with homocysteine stimulating the increased expression of *sterol regulatory element binding proteins* (SREBP), [256] which bind to specific DNA sequences that encode lipid producing enzymes.[257] Other abnormalities have also been observed such as impaired LCAT activity, increased levels of triglycerides and diminished activity of the enzyme thiolase, involved in the beta oxidation of fatty acids.[258] Beta oxidation is part of a process where fatty acids are used for generating ATP (energy) in the mitochondria.

Interestingly however, homocysteine is not necessarily a bad thing. According to Dr. McCully, in small amounts, it is associated with the growth and support of tissue and bone formation. It also activates insulin like growth factor, a protein that behaves like growth hormone,[259] capable of acting as a powerful inhibitor of apoptosis. [260]

In order to control homocysteine levels, metabolism through two pathways must occur: re-methylation back to methionine or removal through trans-sulfuration.[261] Re-methylation involves the use of B12 dependent betaine: homocysteine methyltransferase (BHMT), an enzyme whose tissue distribution is somewhat limited, or the more widely distributed methionine synthase (MS), which requires B12 as a cofactor and 5-methyltetrahydrofolate as the substrate.[262] Removal also involves transsulfuration enzymes cystathionine synthase (CBS) and cystathionine y-lyase (CGL), both of which are dependent upon vitamin B6.[263]

Needless to say, deficiencies of these B vitamins, B12, Folate and B6, are associated with hyperhomocysteinemia. But the presence of various genetic polymorphisms, or unique gene expressions that effect how enzymes function, can also effect homocysteine levels, most notably, with the enzyme methylene tetrahydrofolate reductase (MTHR- C677TT), which has been estimated to effect between 10 and 20% of the population.[264] The presence of this genetic condition may require use of a folic acid supplement or folate in a co-enzymated, or active form such as *methyfolate*.

There are other factors that can affect homocysteine levels. From a nutritional standpoint, there are secondary cofactors that play a role. For example, low levels of riboflavin, especially in those with the MTHFR C677TT phenotype, have been shown to be inversely related to homocysteine levels.[265] Riboflavin, in its coenzyme form FMN, is required by pyridoxine phosphate oxidase for converting B6 to its coenzyme form, pyridoxal phosphate [266], which can effect transsulfuration activity. Zinc status may also play a role in homocysteine levels since its relationship with folylpolyglytamate hydrolase ensures that folate will be absorbed into intestinal cells,[267] thereby assuring proper folate status.

Sub clinical deficiency of vitamin C

The most obvious connection between vitamin C and cholesterol, as previously mentioned, is its ability to act as an antioxidant offering protection from oxidative stress. In fact those who already exhibit hyperlipidemia may be more susceptible to oxidation, requiring higher intakes.[268] But this relationship is not limited to protection from free radical activity. Research as early as 1976, showed the link between vitamin C and its role as a cofactor in cholesterol 7 alpha hydroxylase activity. This biochemical pathway is vital for the production of bile[269], which assists in lowering available cholesterol by using it as a raw material. Vitamin C is also a critical cofactor in the production of L-carnitine. This non-protein nitrogen compound composed of lysine and methionine is involved in fatty acid oxidation and subsequent energy production, and low levels have been linked with low HDL levels in the body.[270],[271]

In research utilizing guinea pigs, it has been shown that vitamin D receptors (VDRs) critical for mediating the physiological function of vitamin D can be reduced in number by deficiencies of vitamin C. [272] Folate or the synthetic form, folic acid, so important in the prevention of homocysteine, appears to rely on vitamin C for utilization. [273], [274] And sub clinical deficiencies of vitamin C have been associated with such pre-scorbutic signs as infection susceptibility. [275] There has been recent research showing the connection between vitamin C status and C-reactive protein (CRP).[276] For vitamin C to be effective at lowering CRP, the baseline CRP levels need to be indicative of an elevated risk for cardiovascular disease. What is significant here is that the effect of vitamin C, at a dose of 1000 mg a day, was similar to that of statin drugs.[277] Low levels of ascorbic acid have also been shown to have an inverse relationship with plasminogen activator -1 or PAI-1, a promoter of coagulation. [278] As previously mentioned, PAI-1 is associated with hyperlipidemia, but its link does not appear to be a direct one. In fact there is research that indicates that PAI-1 is initiated by factors that are both pro-oxidant and pro-inflammatory in nature. But in particular, it has been linked with TNF-alpha, a regulator that controls intensity early on in the inflammatory process.[279]

While several sources link vitamin C and thyroid function, the specific action appears to be unclear. [280], [281] One study with thyroidectimized rats, showed that both tissue and serum levels of vitamin C were decreased. In addition, there was an increase not only in the activity of the hepatic degrading enzyme, involved in the degradation of insulin in the liver[282], but also in the excretion of vitamin C.[283] In guinea pigs, low vitamin C was associated with the deiodination, and since this activity can be involved in activating or inactivating thyroid hormone, there could be interference with the synthesis of both T3 and T4.[284], [285] In addition, poor vitamin C status was also linked with decreases in organification, [286] or the process by which iodide is oxidized and subsequently incorporated into tyrosine residue to form thyroglobulin. Another consideration is the fact that T3 hormones are involved in energy metabolism with the mitochondria, creating a *calorigenic* effect, or an increase in heat or energy. As a result, there is an increase in the consumption of oxygen by T3 leading to an increase in the production of reactive oxygen and nitrogen species.[287] The role of vitamin C in thyroid health, also appears to be involved in the protection of oxidation of the gland.

And finally, there is a stress component indirectly linking lipoprotein levels with vitamin C status. In comparison to other organs and tissues, the adrenal glands contain the highest concentration of vitamin C, which is important since this is the primary site for the synthesis of norepinephrine. [288] It also appears that in order to release adrenal hormones into circulation, ascorbate is needed. [289] In fact there appears to be multiple reactions in this pathway that require vitamin C. Tyrosine may not be completely catabolized when ascorbate is deficient. [290] It is also directly involved in the activity of dopamine-B-hydroxylase necessary in the synthesis of norepinephrine, from dopamine. [291] (Epinephrine is ultimately manufactured when norepinephrine is methylated.)

What this information suggests is that a chronic stress response can have a dramatic effect on the amount and availability of tyrosine which can not only affect the availability of thyroid hormone, but also the ability to synthesize catecholamines dopamine, norepinephrine and epinephrine. These reactions may explain why stress is linked to hyperlipidemia and it is clear that additional study in this area can more fully explain the connection between vitamin C status and normal lipoprotein levels.

Conclusion

We know that cholesterol is an important raw material for manufacturing hormone and hormone-like substances as well as structural components for cell membranes and as a result, is necessary for health and wellbeing. However, cholesterol, as a type of lipid, is not the same thing as Low Density or High Density Lipoproteins (LDL/HDL)-- two lipid transport systems within the body. Distinguishing between cholesterol and lipoproteins is necessary for recognizing that an increase in the transport of lipids and other lipid soluble products may be due to some kind of nutrient imbalance or an increased need for raw materials.

What Causes Elevated Low Density Lipoproteins?

It has been long considered that elevated lipoproteins, particularly low density lipoproteins has been linked to the development of heart disease and that by lowering these levels pharmacologically will help improve patient outcome. But this method is not without side effects and may not positively impact mortality rates. Using a Functional Nutrition model, or how the presence or absence of a substance in a food determines how the body uses that food, it may be possible to determine the multiple nutritional links, deficiencies or excesses that can impact the need for cholesterol and as a result, Low Density Lipoprotein levels.

Since inflammation of an on-going nature appears to be a major link in the development of many chronic degenerative diseases in general and cholesterol homeostasis, in particular, it is important to determine which nutrients are associated with the development or prevention of the inflammatory response. Such nutrients/compounds include: antioxidants, sterols and sterolins, vitamins E, D, C, and B vitamins, as well as certain minerals like magnesium and chromium. Essential fatty acid imbalances, excesses in sugar, are also contributory as are physical activity, high levels of stress, and immune and/or detoxification challenges. Clearly, maintaining proper cholesterol levels and its availability via lipoprotein transport is a complex, interconnecting web of many biochemical variables that requires a more functional approach when attempting to resolve hyperlipidemia.

Endnotes

1   The New York Times http://www.nytimes.com/2008/01/14/business/14cnd-drug.html?em&ex=1200546000&en=3790ea9662bb0e93&ei=5087%0A Accessed February 2, 2008.

2   Jones, David S. Editor in Chief, Textbook of Functional Medicine, Institute For Functional Nutrition, *Gig Harbor*, Wa. 2005, pg, 276.

3   *Liver phases 1 and 2 detoxification pathways,* balancedconcepts.net/liver_phases_detox_paths.pdf, Accessed 5/12/19.

4   Jones, David S., Editor in Chief, Textbook of Functional Medicine, Institute For Functional Nutrition, *Gig Harbor*, Wa. 2005, pg. 641.

5   Shelton, RC, Manning, JS, Barentine, LW, Tipa, EV. *Assessing Effects of l-Methylfolate in Depression Management: Results of a Real-World Patient Experience Trial* Prim Care Companion CNS Disord. 2013; 15(4).

6   Mischoulon D, Raab MF. *The role of folate in depression and dementia.* J Clin Psychiatry. 2007; 68 Suppl 10:28-33.

7   Young, Simon N, *Folate and depression—a neglected problem.* J Psychiatry Neurosci. 2007 March; 32(2): 80–82.

8   The New York Times, http://www.nytimes.com/2008/01/14/business/14cnd-drug.html?em&ex=1200546000&en=3790ea9662bb0e93&ei=5087%0A Accessed February 2, 2008.

9   Jones, PJ, Am J Clin Nutr, Aug 1997, 66(2):438-46.

10 Julias, AD, et al, J Nutr, Dec 1982, 112(12):2240-9).

11 Morell, Pierre, Quarles, Richard H., Characteristic Composition of Myelin Basic Neurochemistry: Molecular, Cellular and Medical Aspects. 6th edition. Siegel GJ, Agranoff BW, Albers RW, et al., editors. Philadelphia: Lippincott-Raven; 1999 https://www.ncbi.nlm.nih.gov/books/NBK28221/

12 Erasmus, Udo, Fats That Heal, Fats That Kill, Alive Books, Burnaby BC Canada V5J5B9, 1997, pg 84.

[13]   MCH Links, USDA/ARS Children's Nutrition Research Center at Baylor College of Medicine. *Cholesterol Content: Another Difference between Human Milk and Infant Formula.* Retrieved November 2, 2007.

[14]   ScienceDirect,   http://www.sciencedirect.com/topics/medicine-and-denstistry/cholesterol-synthesis, accessed 5/12/19.

[15]   Gropper, SS, Smith, JL, Groff, JL. (2005) Advanced Nutrition And Human Metablism. Belmont, Ca. Thomson Wadsworth, pg 160.

[16]   Ibid. pg. 161.

[17]   Erasmus, Udo, Fats That Heal, Fats That Kill, Alive Books, Burnaby BC Canada V5J5B9, 1997, pg. 66.

[18]   Hess, Cathy Thomas, RN, BSN, CWOCN, Clinical Guide: Skin And Wound Care, Sixth Edition, Lippincott, Williams and Wilkins, Ambler Pa., 2008, pg. 5.

[19]   Ibid.

[20]   MCH Links, USDA/ARS Children's Nutrition Research Center at Baylor College of Medicine. *Cholesterol Content: Another Difference between Human Milk and Infant Formula.* Retrieved November 2, 2007.

[21]   Engelberg, H, *Low serum cholesterol and suicide.* Lancet 1992 Mar 21;339(8795):727-9.

[22]   Hawthon K, Cowen P, Owens D, Bond A, Elliott M. *Low serum cholesterol and suicide.* The British Journal of Psychiatry 162: 818-825 (1993).

[23]   Cornell NEWS. *W.M. Keck Foundation gives $1.5 million to start research/training program at Cornell and Weill Medical College to learn how cells communicate.* Retrieved February 26, 2007.

[24]   Cell Communication And Signaling. *7-Ketocholesterol modulates intercellular communication through gap-junction in bovine lens epithelial cells.* Retrieved February 26, 2007.

[25]   Southwestern Medical Center. *Researchers discover a good side to cholesterol in controlling cell signals.* Retrieved February 26, 2007.
       Smith LL. *Another cholesterol hypothesis: cholesterol as antioxidant.* Free Radic Biol Med. 1991;11(1):47-61.

[26]   Zhang W, Demattia JA, Song H, Couldwell WT. *Communication between malignant glioma cells and vascular endothelial cells through gap junctions.* J Neurosurg. 2003 Apr;98(4):846-53.

[27]   G L Nicolson, K M Dulski, and J E Trosko. *Loss of intercellular junctional communication correlates with metastatic potential in mammary adenocarcinoma cells.* Proc Natl Acad Sci U S A. 1988 January; 85(2): 473–476.

28 Medscape Today, http://www.medscape.com/viewarticle/560345?sssdmh=dm1.289174&src=nldne Accessed 7/27/07.

29 Alsheikh-Ali AA, Maddukuri PV, Han H, Karas RH. *Effect of the magnitude of lipid lowering on risk of elevated liver enzymes, rhabdomyolysis, and cancer: insights from large randomized statin trials.* J Am Coll Cardiol. 2007 Jul 31;50(5):409-18. Epub 2007 Jul 16.

30 Albrecht I, Gatfield J, Mini T, Jeno P, Pieters J. *Essential role for cholesterol in the delivery of exogenous antigens to the MHC class I-presentation pathway.* Int Immunol. 2006 May;18(5):755-65. Epub 2006 Apr 11.

31 Rock KL, Shen L. *Cross-presentation: underlying mechanisms and role in immune surveillance.* Immunol Rev. 2005 Oct;207:166-83.

32 Calcagni E, Elenkov I. *Stress system activity, innate and T helper cytokines, and susceptibility to immune-related diseases.* Ann. N.Y. Acad. Sci. 1069: 62–76 (2006).

33 Engstrom G, Hedblad B, Janzon L, Lindgarde F. *Long-term change in cholesterol in relation to inflammation-sensitive plasma proteins: a longitudinal study.* Ann Epidemiol. 2007 Jan;17(1):57-63

34 Beard, JA, Bearden, A, Striker, R. *Vitamin D and the anti-viral state.* J Clin Virol. 2011 Mar; 50(3): 194–200.

35 Wood, WG et al. Lipids, Mar 1999, 34(3):225-234.

36 De Rosa S, Cirillo P, Paglia A, Sasso L, Di Palma V, Chiariello M. *Reactive Oxygen Species and Antioxidants in the Pathophysiology of Cardiovascular Disease: Does the Actual Knowledge Justify a Clinical Approach?* Curr Vasc Pharmacol. 2010 Jan 1. [Epub ahead of print]

37 National Cancer Institute. http://www.cancer.gov/cancertopics/factsheet/prevention/antioxidants Retrieved September 28, 2009.

38 Marieb, EN, Hoen, K, Human Anatomy & Physiology, 8th Edition. Benjamin Cumings, 2010, pg. 769.

39 McCance KL, Huether SE, Pathophysiology: The Biolologic Basis for Disease in Adults and Children, Third Edition. Mosby, NY, 1998, pg. 228.

40 Ibid. pg. 207-208.

41 Ibid. pg. 226.

42 Ibid. pg. 227

43 Ibid. pps. 195-196.

44 Wilkinson I, Cockcroft JR. *Cholesterol, lipids and arterial stiffness.* Adv Cardiol. 2007;44:261-77.

45 Feingold KR, Hardardóttir I, Grunfeld C. *Beneficial effects of cytokine induced hyperlipidemia.* Z Ernahrungswiss. 1998;37 Suppl 1:66-74

[46] http://medical-dictionary.thefreedictionary.com/Apolipoprotein+A1 Accessed 7/18/07

[47] Ancsin J B, Kisilevsky R. The Heparin/Heparan Sulfate-binding Site on Apo-serum Amyloid A IMPLICATIONS FOR THE THERAPEUTIC INTERVENTION OF AMYLOIDOSIS. J Biol Chem, Vol. 274, Issue 11, 7172-7181, March 12, 1999. Accessed 11/25/07.

[48] http://www.medterms.com/script/main/art.asp?articlekey=30788 Accessed 11/25/07.

[49] Zhang N, Ahsan MH, Purchia AF, West DB. *Serum Amyloid A-Luciferase Transgenic Mice: Response to Sepsis, Acute Arthritis, and Contact Hypersensitivity and the Effects of Proteasome Inhibition.* The Journal of Immunology, 174: 8125-8134, 2005. Accessed 7/18/07.

[50] MedicineNet.com http://www.medterms.com/script/main/art.asp?article key=30788 Accessed 11/25/07

[51] Urieli-Shoval S, Linke RP, Matzner Y. *Expression and function of serum amyloid A, a major acute-phase protein, in normal and disease states.* Curr Opin Hematol. 2000 Jan;7(1):64-9.

[52] Feingold KR, Hardardóttir I, Grunfeld C. *Beneficial effects of cytokine induced hyperlipidemia.* Z Ernahrungswiss. 1998;37 Suppl 1:66-74.

[53] Khovidhunkit W, Kim MS, Memon RA, Shigenaga JK, Moser AH, Feingold KR, Grunfeld C. *Effects of infection and inflammation on lipid and lipoprotein metabolism: mechanisms and consequences to the host.* J Lipid Res. 2004 Jul;45(7):1169-96. Epub 2004 Apr 21.

[54] Kaunitz H, *Cholesterol and repair processes in arteriosclerosis.* Lipids1978 May;13(5):373-4.

[55] Pfohl M, Schreiber I, Liebich HM, Häring HU, Hoffmeister HM. *Upregulation of cholesterol synthesis after acute myocardial infarction--is cholesterol a positive acute phase reactant?* Atherosclerosis. 1999 Feb;142(2):389-93.

[56] Esteve E, Ricart W, Fernández-Real JM. *Dyslipidemia and inflammation: an evolutionary conserved mechanism.* Clin Nutr. 2005 Feb;24(1):16-31.

[57] Marieb EN, Human Anatomy & Physiology, 6th Edition, Pearson, Benjamin Cummings, NY, 2004, pg. 789.

[58] Jones, David S., Editor in Chief, Textbook of Functional Medicine, Institute For Functional Nutrition, Gig Harbor, Wa. 2005, pg.190.

[59] IgG vs IgE: What is the difference? **Healthscope Functional Pathology** Practitioner Manual 2011, www.healthscopepathology.com.au/index. php/download_file/view/183/133/

60 McCance KL, Huether SE, Pathophysiology: <u>The Biolologic Basis for Disease in Adults and Children, Third Edition</u>. Mosby, NY, 1998, pg. 205.

61 Biology-Online.org http://www.biology-online.org/dictionary/Endotoxin Accessed 7/21/07

62 Answers.com http://www.answers.com/topic/endotoxin Accessed 7/21/07

63 Stoll LL, Denning GM, Weintraub NL. *Endotoxin, TLR4 signaling and vascular inflammation: potential therapeutic targets in cardiovascular disease.* Curr Pharm Des. 2006;12(32):4229-45.

64 Cell Signaling Technology http://www.cellsignal.com/reference/kinase/ Accessed 8/11/09.

65 Cheng Q, Cant CA, Moll T, Hofer-Warbinek R, Wagner E, Birnstiel ML, Bach FH, de Martin R. *NK-kappa B subunit-specific regulation of the I kappa B alpha promoter.* J Biol Chem. 1994 May 6;269(18):13551-7.

66 Favier A. *[Oxidative stress in human diseases]* Ann Pharm Fr. 2006 Nov;64(6):390-6.

67 Singh U, Jialal I. *Oxidative stress and atherosclerosis.* Pathophysiology. 2006 Aug;13(3):129-42. Epub 2006 Jun 6.

68 Madamanchi NR, Vendrov A, Runge MS. *Oxidative stress and vascular disease.* Arterioscler Thromb Vasc Biol. 2005 Jan;25(1):29-38. Epub 2004 Nov 11.

69 Parthasarathy S, Santanam N, Ramachandran S, Meilhac O. *Potential role of oxidized lipids and lipoproteins in antioxidant defense.* Free Radic Res. 2000 Sep;33(3):197-215.

70 Sinatra, Stephen, MD, FACC, FACN, Sinatra, Jan, MSN, CNS, APRN, *Lower Your Blood Pressure in Eight Weeks,* Ballantine Books, NY 2003, pps. 59.

71 Dirican M, Serdar Z, Sarandol E, Surmen-Gur E, Lecithin:Cholesterol Acyltransferace Activity And Cholesterol Ester Transfer Rate In Patients With Diabetes Mellitus. Turk J Med Sci 33:95-101, 2003.

72 JK Bielicki, TM Forte and MR McCall. *Minimally oxidized LDL is a potent inhibitor of lecithin:cholesterol acyltransferase activity.* Journal of Lipid Research, Vol 37, 1012-1021, 1996.

73 Moore RE, Navab M, Millar JS, Zimetti F, Hama S, Rothblat GH, Rader DJ. *Increased atherosclerosis in mice lacking apolipoprotein A-I attributable to both impaired reverse cholesterol transport and increased inflammation.* Circ Res. 2005 Oct 14;97(8):763-71. Epub 2005 Sep 8.

[74] Shao B, Oda MN, Vaisar T, Oram JF, Heinecke JW. *Pathways for oxidation of high-density lipoprotein in human cardiovascular disease.* Curr Opin Mol Ther. 2006 Jun;8(3):198-205.

[75] Uchino BN, Holt-Lunstad J, Bloor LE, Campo RA. *Aging and cardiovascular reactivity to stress: longitudinal evidence for changes in stress reactivity.* Psychol Aging. 2005 Mar;20(1):134-43.

[76] Colbin, A, PhD., *The Cholesterol Controversy.* The Journal Alternative & Complementary Therapies, vol 11 No. 3, June 2005, pp 126-30.

[77] Black PH, Garbutt LD. *Stress, inflammation and cardiovascular disease.* J Psychosom Res. 2002 Jan;52(1):1-23.

[78] Ibid.

[79] McEwen BS. *Protective and damaging effects of stress mediators: central role of the brain.* Dialogues Clin Neurosci. 2006;8(4):367-81.

[80] Jones, David S., Editor in Chief, <u>Textbook of Functional Medicine,</u> <u>Institute For Functional Nutrition,</u> Gig Harbor, Wa. 2005, pg. 670.

[81] Schulz KH, Heesen C, Gold SM. *[The concept of allostasis and allostatic load: psychoneuroimmunological findings]* Psychother Psychosom Med Psychol. 2005 Nov;55(11):452-61.

[82] McEwen BS. *Allostasis and allostatic load: implications for neuropsychopharmacology.* Neuropsychopharmacology. 2000 Feb;22(2):108-24.

[83] Ibid.

[84] Scott M. Grundy, MD, PhD; H. Bryan Brewer, Jr, MD; James I. Cleeman, MD; Sidney C. Smith, Jr, MD; Claude Lenfant, MD, for the Conference Participants, *Definition of Metabolic Syndrome,* NHLBI/AHA Conference Proceedings, *Circulation.* 2004;109:433-438.

[85] Abraham NG, Brunner EJ, Eriksson JW, Robertson RP. *Metabolic Syndrome: Psychosocial, Neuroendocrine and Classical Risk Factors in Type 2 Diabetes.* Ann N Y Acad Sci. 2007 May 18; [Epub ahead of print]

[86] MedicinNet.com. http://www.medterms.com/script/main/art.asp?articlekey=25458 Accessed 7/19/07.

[87] Ishikawa K, Takahashi K, Bujo H, Hashimoto N, Yagui K, Saito Y. *Subcutaneous fat modulates insulin sensitivity in mice by regulating TNF-alpha expression in visceral fat.* Horm Metab Res. 2006 Oct;38(10):631-8.

[88] Bhatheja R, Bhatt DL. *Clinical outcomes in metabolic syndrome.* J Cardiovasc Nurs. 2006 Jul-Aug;21(4):298-305.

[89] Frassetto L, Morris RC Jr, Sellmeyer DE, Todd K, Sebastian A. *Diet, evolution and aging--the pathophysiologic effects of the post-agricultural*

inversion of the potassium-to-sodium and base-to-chloride ratios in the human diet. Eur J Nutr. 2001 Oct;40(5):200-13.

90 Eaton SB. *The ancestral human diet: what was it and should it be a paradigm for contemporary nutrition?* Proc Nutr Soc. 2006 Feb;65(1):1-6.

91 Cordain L, Eaton SB, Sebastian A, Mann N, Lindeberg S, Watkins BA, O'Keefe JH, Brand-Miller J. *Origins and evolution of the Western diet: health implications for the 21st century,* American Journal of Clinical Nutrition, Vol. 81, No. 2, 341-354, February 2005.

92 Sebastian A, Frassetto LA, Sellmeyer DE, Merriam RL, Morris RC. *Estimation of the net acid load of the diet of ancestral preagricultural Homo sapiens and their hominid ancestors.* Am J Clin Nutr 2002;76:1308-16.

93 Feldeisen SE, Tucker KL. *Nutritional strategies in the prevention and treatment of metabolic syndrome.* Appl Physiol Nutr Metab. 2007 Feb;32(1):46-60.

94 Geiss HC, Parhofer K. *[Diabetic dyslipoproteinemia]* MMW Fortschr Med. 2006 Apr 6;148(14):30-3.

95 Nesto RW. Beyond low-density lipoprotein: addressing the atherogenic lipid triad in type 2 diabetes mellitus and the metabolic syndrome. Am J Cardiovasc Drugs. 2005;5(6):379-87.

96 Mitch WE. *Metabolic and clinical consequences of metabolic acidosis.* J Nephrol. 2006 Mar-Apr;19 Suppl 9:S70-5.

97 Brungger M, Hulter HN, Krapf R. *Effect of chronic metabolic acidosis on thyroid hormone homeostasis in humans.* Am J Physiol. 1997 May;272(5 Pt 2):F648-53.

98 Ibid.

99 Aso Y, Wakabayashi S, Yamamoto R, Matsutomo R, Takebayashi K, Inukai T. *Metabolic syndrome accompanied by hypercholesterolemia is strongly associated with proinflammatory state and impairment of fibrinolysis in patients with type 2 diabetes: synergistic effects of plasminogen activator inhibitor-1 and thrombin-activatable fibrinolysis inhibitor.* Diabetes Care. 2005 Sep;28(9):2211-6.

100 Georgieva AM, Cate HT, Keulen ET, van Oerle R, Govers-Riemslag JW, Hamulyak K, van der Kallen CJ, Van Greevenbroek MM, De Bruin TW. *Prothrombotic markers in familial combined hyperlipidemia: evidence of endothelial cell activation and relation to metabolic syndrome. Atherosclerosis.* 2004 Aug;175(2):345-51.

101 Assaf, Areej M., Al-Abbassi, Reem, Al-Binni, Mayasaa. *Academic stress-induced changes in Th1- and Th2-cytokine response.* Saudi Pharm J. 2017 Dec; 25(8): 1237–1247.

[102] Suter PM. *Carbohydrates and dietary fiber.* Handb Exp Pharmacol. 2005;(170):231-61.

[103] Ludwig DS. *Diet and development of the insulin resistance syndrome.* Asia Pac J Clin Nutr. 2003;12 Suppl:S4.

[104] Qi L, van Dam RM, Liu S, Franz M, Mantzoros C, Hu FB. *Whole-grain, bran, and cereal fiber intakes and markers of systemic inflammation in diabetic women.* Diabetes Care. 2006 Feb;29(2):207-11.

[105] Wu T, Giovannucci E, Pischon T, Hankinson SE, Ma J, Rifai N, Rimm EB. *Fructose, glycemic load, and quantity and quality of carbohydrate in relation to plasma C-peptide concentrations in US women.* Am J Clin Nutr. 2004 Oct;80(4):1043-9.

[106] Kelley GL, Allan G, Azhar S. *High dietary fructose induces a hepatic stress response resulting in cholesterol and lipid dysregulation.* Endocrinology. 2004 Feb;145(2):548-55. Epub 2003 Oct 23.

[107] Busserolles J, Rock E, Gueux E, Mazur A, Grolier P, Rayssiguier Y. *Short-term consumption of a high-sucrose diet has a pro-oxidant effect in rats.* Br J Nutr. 2002 Apr;87(4):337-42.

[108] Busserolles J, Gueux E, Rock E, Mazur A, Rayssiguier Y. *High fructose feeding of magnesium deficient rats is associated with increased plasma triglyceride concentration and increased oxidative stress.* Magnes Res. 2003 Mar;16(1):7-12

[109] Jones, David S., Editor in Chief, <u>Textbook of Functional Medicine, Institute For Functional Nutrition,</u> Gig Harbor, Wa. 2005, pg. 383.

[110] van Buul, Vincent J, Tappy, Luc, and Brouns, Frederick JPH. *Misconceptions about fructose-containing sugars and their role in the obesity epidemic.* Nutr Res Rev. 2014 Jun; 27(1): 119–130.

[111] *Peroxisome Proliferator-Activated Receptors, PPARs.* <u>https://themedical biochemistrypage.org/ppar.php.</u> Accessed 1/20/18.

[112] Bland, JS. *The Fructose Controversy: Separating Fact from Fiction.* JANA, Vol. 8, No. 3, 2005, pg.3.

[113] Basciano H, Federico L, Adeli K. *Fructose, insulin resistance, and metabolic dyslipidemia.* Nutr Metab (Lond). 2005 Feb 21;2(1):5.

[114] Elliott SS, Keim NL, Stern JS, Teff K, Havel PJ. *Fructose, weight gain, and the insulin resistance syndrome.* Am J Clin Nutr. 2002 Nov;76(5):911-22.

[115] Zawn Villines, Reviewed by Katherine Marengo, LDN, RD. "What foods contain high fructose corn sweetener?" *Medical News Today,* Last reviewed Wed 29 May 2019, <u>https://www.medicalnewstoday.com/articles/325315.php</u>

[116] Ibid.

[117] Alesci S, Martinez PE, Kelkar S, Ilias I, Ronsaville DS, Listwak SJ, Ayala AR, Licinio J, Gold HK, Kling MA, Chrousos GP, Gold PW. *Major depression is associated with significant diurnal elevations in plasma interleukin-6 levels, a shift of its circadian rhythm, and loss of physiological complexity in its secretion: ngclinical implications.* J Clin Endocrinol Metab. 2005 May;90(5):2522-30. Epub 2005 Feb 10.

[118] Endotox.com http://www.endotext.org/obesity/obesity12/obesityframe 12.htm Accessed 8/02/09.

[119] Wiecek A, Kokot F, Chudek J, Adamczak M. *The adipose tissue--a novel endocrine organ of interest to the nephrologist.* Nephrol Dial Transplant. 2002 Feb;17(2):191-5.

[120] Andersson CX, Sopasakis VR, Wallerstedt E, Smith U. *Insulin antagonizes interleukin-6 signaling and is anti-inflammatory in 3T3-L1 adipocytes.* J Biol Chem. 2007 Mar 30;282(13):9430-5. Epub 2007 Jan 31.

[121] Dandona P, Aljada A, Bandyopadhyay A. *Inflammation: the link between insulin resistance, obesity and diabetes.* Trends Immunol. 2004 Jan;25(1):4-7.

[122] de Alvaro C, Teruel T, Hernandez R, Lorenzo M. *Tumor necrosis factor alpha produces insulin resistance in skeletal muscle by activation of inhibitor kappaB kinase in a p38 MAPK-dependent manner.* J Biol Chem. 2004 Apr 23;279(17):17070-8. Epub 2004 Feb 4.

[123] Eckel, Juergen. "Adipose Tissue." Science Direct. 2018. https://www.sciencedirect.com/topics/neuroscience/adipokine accessed 7/9/19.

[124] Guerre-Millo M. *Adipose tissue secretory function: implication in metabolic and cardiovascular complications of obesity.* J Soc Biol. 2006;200(1):37-43.

[125] Xavier Pi-Sunyer F. *The relation of adipose tissue to cardiometabolic risk.* Clin Cornerstone. 2006;8 Suppl 4:S14-23.

[126] Krysiak R, Okopien B, Herman ZS. *[Adipose tissue: a new endocrine organ]* Przegl Lek. 2005;62(9):919-23.

[127] Rector RS, Warner SO, Liu Y, Hinton PS, Sun G, Cox RH, Stump CS, Laughlin MH, Dellsperger KC, Thomas TR. *Exercise and diet induced weight loss improves measures of oxidative stress and insulin sensitivity in adults with characteristics of the metabolic syndrome.* Am J Physiol Endocrinol Metab. 2007 May 1; [Epub ahead of print]

[128] Bastard JP, Maachi M, Lagathu C, Kim MJ, Caron M, Vidal H, Capeau J, Feve B. *Recent advances in the relationship between obesity, inflammation, and insulin resistance.* Eur Cytokine Netw. 2006 Mar;17(1):4-12.

[129] Huypens P. *Adipokines regulate systemic insulin sensitivity in accordance to existing energy reserves.* Med Hypotheses. 2007 Jan 5; [Epub ahead of print]

[130] Calvani M, Scarfone A, Granato L, Mora EV, Nanni G, Castagneto M, Greco AV, Manco M, Mingrone G. *Restoration of adiponectin pulsatility in severely obese subjects after weight loss.* Diabetes. 2004 Apr;53(4):939-47.

[131] Wannamethee SG, Whincup PH, Lennon L, Sattar N. *Circulating adiponectin levels and mortality in elderly men with and without cardiovascular disease and heart failure.* Arch Intern Med. 2007 Jul 23;167(14):1510-7.

[132] Varady KA, Lamarche B, Santosa S, Demonty I, Charest A, Jones PJ. *Effect of weight loss resulting from a combined low-fat diet/exercise regimen on low-density lipoprotein particle size and distribution in obese women.* Metabolism. 2006 Oct;55(10):1302-7.

[133] Pasanisi F, Contaldo F, de Simone G, Mancini M. *Benefits of sustained moderate weight loss in obesity.* Nutr Metab Cardiovasc Dis. 2001 Dec;11(6):401-6.

[134] Basciano H, Federico L, Adeli K, *Fructose, insulin resistance, and metabolic dyslipidemia.* Nutr Metab (Lond). 2005 Feb 21;2(1):5.

[135] Tappy L, Lê KA. *Metabolic effects of fructose and the worldwide increase in obesity.* Physiol Rev. 2010 Jan;90(1):23-46.

[136] Faeh D, Minehira K, Schwarz JM, Periasamy R, Park S, Tappy L. *Effect of fructose overfeeding and fish oil administration on hepatic de novo lipogenesis and insulin sensitivity in healthy men.* Diabetes. 2005 Jul;54(7):1907-13.

[137] Howard BV, Wylie-Rosett J. *Circulation: Journal of the Am. Heart Assoc. Sugar and Cardiovascular Disease: A Statement for Health Care Professionals From the Committee on Nutrition, Physical Activity, and Metabolism of the Heart Association. Circulation* 2002; 106;526.

[138] IBID.

[139] MedicineNet.com http://www.medterms.com/script/main/art.asp?articlekey=18822 Accessed 6/20/07.

[140] Nakanishi N, Shiraishi T, Wada M. *Association between C-reactive protein and insulin resistance in a Japanese population: the Minoh Study.* Intern Med. 2005 Jun;44(6):542-7.

[141] Park SH, Kim BI, Yun JW, Kim JW, Park DI, Cho YK, Sung IK, Park CY, Sohn CI, Jeon WK, Kim H, Rhee EJ, Lee WY, Kim SW. *Insulin resistance and C-reactive protein as independent risk factors for non-alcoholic fatty liver disease in non-obese Asian men.* J Gastroenterol Hepatol. 2004 Jun;19(6):694-8.

142 Ucak S, Ekmekci TR, Basat O, Koslu A, Altuntas Y. *Comparison of various insulin sensitivity indices in psoriatic patients and their relationship with type of psoriasis.* J Eur Acad Dermatol Venereol. 2006 May;20(5):517-22.

143 Kanauchi M, Kanauchi K, Hashimoto T, Saito Y. *Metabolic syndrome and new category 'pre-hypertension' in a Japanese population.* Curr Med Res Opin. 2004 Sep;20(9):1365-70.

144 Park SH, Kim BI, Yun JW, Kim JW, Park DI, Cho YK, Sung IK, Park CY, Sohn CI, Jeon WK, Kim H, Rhee EJ, Lee WY, Kim SW. *Insulin resistance and C-reactive protein as independent risk factors for non-alcoholic fatty liver disease in non-obese Asian men.* J Gastroenterol Hepatol. 2004 Jun;19(6):694-8.

145 Gropper SS, Smith JL, Groff JL, <u>Advanced Nutrition and Human Metabolism, 4th Edition,</u> Thomson Wadsworth, USA, pg. 463.

146 [No authors listed] *A scientific review: the role of chromium in insulin resistance.* Diabetes Educ. 2004;Suppl:2-14.

147 Roussel AM, Andriollo-Sanchez M, Ferry M, Bryden NA, Anderson RA. *Food chromium content, dietary chromium intake and related biological variables in French free-living elderly.* Br J Nutr. 2007 Aug;98(2):326-31. Epub 2007 Apr 3.

148 Russell RM. *Factors in aging that effect the bioavailability of nutrients.* J Nutr. 2001 Apr;131(4 Suppl):1359S-61S.

149 Vincent JB. *Recent advances in the nutritional biochemistry of trivalent chromium.* Proc Nutr Soc. 2004 Feb;63(1):41-7.

150 Racek J. *[Chromium as an essential element]* Cas Lek Cesk. 2003;142(6):335-9.

151 Cefalu WT, Hu FB. *Role of chromium in human health and in diabetes.* Diabetes Care. 2004 Nov;27(11):2741-51.

152 Rondinone CM, Kramer D. *Proteasome inhibitors regulate tyrosine phosphorylation of IRS-1 and insulin signaling in adipocytes.* Biochem Biophys Res Commun. 2002 Sep 6;296(5):1257-63.

153 Cefalu WT, Hu FB. *Role of chromium in human health and in diabetes.* Diabetes Care. 2004 Nov;27(11):2741-51.

154 Valk EE, Hornstra G. *Relationship between vitamin E requirement and polyunsaturated fatty acid intake in man: a review.* Int J Vitam Nutr Res. 2000 Mar;70(2):31-42.

155 Eitenmiller, Ronald Ray, Lee, Junsoo. <u>Vitamin E: food chemistry, composition and analysis.</u> Marcel Dekker, Inc, Basel, Switzerland, 2004. pg.271.

156 Overview of the Science of Whole Grains http://www.wholegrainscouncil.org/files/ConfScienceReport.pdf, accessed 1/20/09.

157 Stargrove, M.B., Treasure, J., McKee, D.L. (2008) *Herb, Nutrient, and Drug Interactions: Clinical Implications and Therapeutic Strategies,* Elsevier Health Sciences, St. Louis, Mo. Pg. 425

158 Munteanu A, Zingg JM, Azzi A. *Anti-atherosclerotic effects of vitamin E--myth or reality?* J Cell Mol Med. 2004 Jan-Mar;8(1):59-76.

159 Jiang Q, Ames BN. *Gamma-tocopherol, but not alpha-tocopherol, decreases proinflammatory eicosanoids and inflammation damage in rats.* FASEB J. 2003 May;17(8):816-22

160 Gaby, Alan R., *Does High Dose Vitamin E kill people?,* Townsend Letter for Doctors and Patients, Feb-Mar 2005, pps, 259-260.

161 Huang HY, Appel LJ. *Supplementation of diets with alpha-tocopherol reduces serum concentrations of gamma- and delta-tocopherol in humans.* J Nutr 2003;133:3137-3140.

162 Chiu KC, Chu A, Go VL, Saad MF. *Hypovitaminosis D is associated with insulin resistance and beta cell dysfunction.* Am J Clin Nutr. 2004 May;79(5):820-5.

163 Ford ES, Ajani UA, McGuire LC, Liu S. *Concentrations of serum vitamin D and the metabolic syndrome among U.S. adults.* Diabetes Care. 2005 May;28(5):1228-30.

164 Kamycheva E, Jorde R, Figenschau Y, Haug E. *Insulin sensitivity in subjects with secondary hyperparathyroidism and the effect of a low serum 25-hydroxyvitamin D level on insulin sensitivity.* J Endocrinol Invest. 2007 Feb;30(2):126-32.

165 Maghbooli Z, Hossein-Nezhad A, Karimi F, Shafaei AR, Larijani B. *Correlation between vitamin D(3) deficiency and insulin resistance in pregnancy.* Diabetes Metab Res Rev. 2007 Jul 2; [Epub ahead of print]

166 Bodnar LM, Catov JM, Simhan HN, Holick MF, Powers RW, Roberts JM. *Maternal vitamin d deficiency increases the risk of preeclampsia.* J Clin Endocrinol Metab. 2007 Sep;92(9):3517-22. Epub 2007 May 29.

167 Wolf M, Sandler L, Muñoz K, Hsu K, Ecker JL, Thadhani R. *First trimester insulin resistance and subsequent preeclampsia: a prospective study.* J Clin Endocrinol Metab. 2002 Apr;87(4):1563-8.

168 Mathieu C, Gysemans C, Giulietti A, Bouillon R. *Vitamin D and diabetes.* Diabetologia. 2005 Jul;48(7):1247-57. Epub 2005 Jun 22.

169 Smotkin-Tangorra M, Purushothaman R, Gupta A, Nejati G, Anhalt H, Ten S. *Prevalence of vitamin D insufficiency in obese children and adolescents.* J Pediatr Endocrinol Metab. 2007 Jul;20(7):817-23.

170 Holick MF. *The vitamin D epidemic and its health consequences.* J Nutr. 2005 Nov;135(11):2739S-48S.

171 Holick MF, MD, PhD, *Sunlight and Vitamin D, Both Good for Cardiovascular Health* J Gen Intern Med. 2002 September; 17(9): 733–735.

172 OSU Oregon State University http://lpi.oregonstate.edu/infocenter/vitamins/vitaminD/index.html, Accessed 10/09/07.

173 Office of Dietary Supplements http://ods.od.nih.gov/factsheets/vitamind.asp, Accessed 10/09/07.

174 Bao BY, Ting HJ, Hsu JW, Lee YF. *Protective role of 1 alpha, 25-dihydroxyvitamin D3 against oxidative stress in nonmalignant human prostate epithelial cells.* Int J Cancer. 2008 Jun 15;122(12):2699-706.

175 McDowall, Jennifer. (October, 2006). *Cytochrome P450.* RCSB PDB, Retrieved from: https://www.ebi.ac.uk/interpro/potm/2006_10/Page1.htm

176 Wietrzyk J. [3 *The influence of isoflavonoids on the antitumor activity of vitamin D*] Postepy Hig Med Dosw (Online). 2007;61:253-60.

177 OSU Oregon State University http://lpi.oregonstate.edu/infocenter/vitamins/vitaminD/, Accessed 10/ 8/07.

178 Shea, M. Kyla, Holden, Rachel M, Vitamin K Status and Vascular Calcification: Evidence from Observational and Clinical Studies, Adv Nutr. 2012 Mar; 3(2): 158–165.

179 Mercola, J, The Real RDA for Vitamin D is 10 Times Higher Than Currently Recommended, 5/10/15 http://articles.mercola.com/sites/articles/archive/2015/05/10/vitamin-d-recommended-dietary-allowance.aspx

180 182 Institute of Medicine of the National Academies, Dietary Reference Intakes for Calcium and Vitamin D, Revised March 2011 https://www.nationalacademies.org/hmd/~/media/Files/Report%20Files/2010/Dietary-Reference-Intakes-for-Calcium-and-Vitamin-D/Vitamin%20D%20and%20Calcium%202010%20Report%20Brief.pd

181 National Institutes of Health, Vitamin D: Fact sheet for Health Professionals, 2/11/16 http://ods.od.nih.gov/factsheets/vitamind/

182 NCBI http://www.ncbi.nlm.nih.gov/disease/Obesity.html Accessed 6/21/07

183 Marzulo P, Verti B, Savia G, Walke, GE, Guzzaloni G, Tagliarferri M, Di Blasio A, Liuzzo A, *The Relationship between Active Ghrelin Levels and Human Obesity Involves Alterations in Resting Energy Expenditure.* The Journal of Clinical Endocrinology & Metabolism 2004; 89(2):936–939

[184] Copinschi G. *Metabolic and endocrine effects of sleep deprivation.* Essent Psychopharmacol. 2005;6(6):341-7.

[185] Spiege, K, Knutson K, Leproult R, Tasali E, Van Cauter E. *Sleep loss: a novel risk factor for insulin resistance and Typ e 2 diabetes.* J Appl Physiol 99: 2008-2019, 2005; doi:10.1152/japplphysiol.00660.2005.

[186] Irwin MR, Wang M, Campomayor CO, Collado-Hidalgo A, Cole S. *Sleep deprivation and activation of morning levels of cellular and genomic markers of inflammation.* Arch Intern Med. 2006 Sep 18;166(16):1756-62.

[187] Rayssiguier Y, Mazur A. *[Magnesium and inflammation: lessons from animal models]* Clin Calcium. 2005 Feb;15(2):245-8.

[188] Mazur A, Maier JA, Rock E, Gueux E, Nowacki W, Rayssiguier Y. *Magnesium and the inflammatory response: potential physiopathological implications.* Arch Biochem Biophys. 2007 Feb 1;458(1):48-56. Epub 2006 Apr 19.

[189] The Free Dictionary http://encyclopedia.thefreedictionary.com/Acute+phase+proteins Accessed 6/27/07

[190] Ibid.

[191] Hans CP, Chaudhary DP, Bansal DD. *Magnesium deficiency increases oxidative stress in rats.* Indian J Exp Biol. 2002 Nov;40(11):1275-9.

[192] Kuzniar A, Mitura P, Kurys P, Szymonik-Lesiuk S, Florianczyk B, Stryjecka-Zimmer M. *The influence of hypomagnesemia on erythrocyte antioxidant enzyme defence system in mice.* Biometals. 2003 Jun;16(2):349-57.

[193] Hans CP, Sialy R, Bansal DD, *Magnesium deficiency and diabetes mellitus.* Current Science, 2002 Dec; VOL. 83, NO. 12.

[194] Takaya J, Higashino H, Kobayashi Y. *Intracellular magnesium and insulin resistance.* Magnes Res. 2004 Jun;17(2):126-36.

[195] Bara M, Guiet-Bara A. *Magnesium regulation of Ca2+ channels in smooth muscle and endothelial cells of human allantochorial placental vessels.* Magnes Res. 2001 Mar;14(1-2):11-8.

[196] Kisters K, Wessels F, Tokmak F, Krefting ER, Gremmler B, Kosch M, Hausberg M. *Early-onset increased calcium and decreased magnesium concentrations and an increased calcium/magnesium ratio in SHR versus WKY.* Magnes Res. 2004 Dec;17(4):264-9.

[197] Barbagallo M, Dominguez LJ, Galioto A, Ferlisi A, Cani C, Malfa L, Pineo A, Busardo' A, Paolisso G. *Role of magnesium in insulin action, diabetes and cardio-metabolic syndrome X.* Mol Aspects Med. 2003 Feb-Jun;24(1-3):39-52.

[198] Durlach J, Pagès N, Bac P, Bara M, Guiet-Bara A, Agrapart C. *Chronopathological forms of magnesium depletion with hypofunction or with hyperfunction of the biological clock. Magnes Res 2002 Dec; 15(3-4):263-8.*

[199] Rylander R, Remer T, Berkemeyer S, Vormann J. *Acid-base status affects renal magnesium losses in healthy, elderly persons.* J Nutr. 2006 Sep;136(9):2374-7.

[200] Science Daily http://www.sciencedaily.com/releases/2007/04/07041 7182847.htm Accessed 6/27/07

[201] Erasmus, Udo, <u>Fats That Heal, Fats That Kill,</u> Alive Books, Burnaby BC Canada V5J5B9, 1997, pg. 53.

[202] Ibid.

[203] Simopoulos AP. *Human requirement for N-3 polyunsaturated fatty acids.* Poult Sci. 2000 Jul;79(7):961-70.

[204] Science Daily http://www.sciencedaily.com/releases/2007/04/07041 7182847.htm accessed 7/04/07.

[205] Ponnampalam EN, Mann NJ, Sinclair AJ. *Effect of feeding systems on omega-3 fatty acids, conjugated linoleic acid and trans fatty acids in Australian beef cuts: potential impact on human health.* Asia Pac J Clin Nutr. 2006;15(1):21-9.

[206] Rule DC, Broughton KS, Shellito SM, Maiorano G. *Comparison of muscle fatty acid profiles and cholesterol concentrations of bison, beef cattle, elk, and chicken.* J Anim Sci. 2002 May;80(5):1202-11.

[207] Medscape Medical Newshttp://www.medscape.com/viewarticle/555736? iss Accessed 7/04/07.

[208] Erasmus, Udo, <u>Fats That Heal, Fats That Kill,</u> Alive Books, Burnaby BC Canada V5J5B9, 1997, pg. 278.

[209] Pérez-Matute P, Pérez-Echarri N, Martínez JA, Marti A, Moreno-Aliaga MJ. *Eicosapentaenoic acid actions on adiposity and insulin resistance in control and high-fat-fed rats: role of apoptosis, adiponectin and tumour necrosis factor-alpha.* Br J Nutr. 2007 Feb;97(2):389-98.

[210] Haluzik MM, Lacinova Z, Dolinkova M, Haluzikova D, Housa D, Horinek A, Vernerova Z, Kumstyrova T, Haluzik M. *Improvement of insulin sensitivity after peroxisome proliferator-activated receptor-alpha agonist treatment is accompanied by paradoxical increase of circulating resistin levels.* Endocrinology. 2006 Sep;147(9):4517-24. Epub 2006 Jun 1

[211] Goto T, Takahashi N, Kato S, Egawa K, Ebisu S, Moriyama T, Fushiki T, Kawada T. *Phytol directly activates peroxisome proliferator-activated receptor alpha (PPARalpha) and regulates gene expression involved in lipid*

metabolism in PPARalpha-expressing HepG2 hepatocytes. Biochem Biophys Res Commun. 2005 Nov 18;337(2):440-5. Epub 2005 Sep 21.

212 Zhao G, Etherton TD, Martin KR, Gillies PJ, West SG, Kris-Etherton PM. *Dietary alpha-linolenic acid inhibits proinflammatory cytokine production by peripheral blood mononuclear cells in hypercholesterolemic subjects.* Am J Clin Nutr. 2007 Feb;85(2):385-91.

213 Nettleton JA, Katz R. *n-3 long-chain polyunsaturated fatty acids in type 2 diabetes: a review.* J Am Diet Assoc. 2005 Mar;105(3):428-40.

214 Ebbesson SO, Risica PM, Ebbesson LO, Kennish JM, Tejero ME. *Omega-3 fatty acids improve glucose tolerance and components of the metabolic syndrome in Alaskan Eskimos: the Alaska Siberia project.* Int J Circumpolar Health. 2005 Sep;64(4):396-408.

215 Erasmus, Udo, Fats That Heal, Fats That Kill, Alive Books, Burnaby BC Canada V5J5B9, 1997, pg. 51.

216 FoodProcessing.com http://www.foodprocessing.com/vendors/products/2005/165.html Accessed 10/14/07.

217 Brownfiel AG News for America http://www.brownfieldnetwork.com/gestalt/go.cfm?objectid=678C52A7-E2D3-A286-DB675B34A4A6BDBA Accessed 10/14/07.

218 Matt Mullein http://mattmullen.blogspot.com/2005/12/not-enough-low-lin-oil.html Accessed 10/14/07.

219 Illinois Soybean Association. http://www.ilsoy.org/soy-news/article/?id=97 Accessed 10/140/07.

220 Canola Canada, Canola Council of Canada http://www.canola-council.org/performance1-3/performance1-3_2.html Accessed 10/14/07.

221 American Heart Association http://www.americanheart.org/presenter.jhtml?identifier=4632 Accessed 10/14/07.

222 Dr. Ronald Hoffman, http://www.drhoffman.com/page.cfm/216 Accessed 6/28/09.

223 Coulston, AM, Boushey, CJ. Nutrition in the Prevention and Treatment of Disease, Second Edition. Elsevier, New York, pg. 533.

224 Ibid.

225 Ibid.

226 Dr. Ronald Hoffman, http://www.drhoffman.com/page.cfm/216 Accessed 6/28/09.

227 Bouic PJD, Lamprecht JH, *Plant Sterols and Sterolins: A Review of Their Immune-Modulating Properties.* Curr Opin Clin Nutr Metab Care 2001; 4,471-475.

228   Dr. Ronald Hoffman, http://www.drhoffman.com/page.cfm/216 Accessed 6/28/09.

229   Vanderhaeghe LR, Bouic PJD. The Immune System Cure. Kensington Publishing Corp., New York, 1999, pg. 47.

230   Mann GV. *Metabolic consequences of dietary trans fatty acids.* Lancet. 1994 May 21;343(8908):1268-71.

231   Booyens J, van der Merwe CF, *Margarines and coronary artery disease.* Med Hypotheses. 1992 Apr;37(4):241-4.

232   Katan MB, Mensink R, Van Tol A, Zock PL, *Dietary trans fatty acids and their impact on plasma lipoproteins.* Can J Cardiol. 1995 Oct;11 Suppl G:36G-38G.

233   Costa AG, Bressan J, Sabarense CM. *[Trans fatty acids: foods and effects on health]* Arch Latinoam Nutr. 2006 Mar;56(1):12-21.

234   Ascherio A. *Trans fatty acids and blood lipids.* Atheroscler Suppl. 2006 May;7(2):25-7. Epub 2006 May 19.

235   AlerChek, Inc. http://www.alerchek.com/coronaryArteryDisease.htm Accessed 7/12/08

236   Mozaffarian D, Katan MB, Ascherio A, Stampfer MJ, Willett WC. *Trans fatty acids and cardiovascular disease.* N Engl J Med. 2006 Apr 13;354(15):1601-13.

237   Enig, Mary G., *Know Your Fats: The Complete Primer for Understanding the Nutrition of Fats, Oils, and Cholesterol.* Bethesda Press, 2000, pg. 85.

238   Cassagno N, Palos-Pinto A, Costet P, Breilh D, Darmon M, Bérard AM. *Low amounts of trans 18:1 fatty acids elevate plasma triacylglycerols but not cholesterol and alter the cellular defence to oxidative stress in mice.* Br J Nutr. 2005 Sep;94(3):346-52.

239   Rise'rus U. Uppsala University, Sweden. *Trans fatty acids, insulin sensitivity and type 2 diabetes.* Scandinavian Journal of Food and Nutrition 2006; 50 (4): 161 _165.

240   Smith U, Kahn BB. *Adipose tissue regulates insulin sensitivity: role of adipogenesis, de novo lipogenesis and novel lipds.* J Intern Med. 2016 Nov;280(5):465-475.

241   Osso FS, Moreira AS, Teixeira MT, Pereira RO, Tavares do Carmo MG, Moura AS. *Trans fatty acids in maternal milk lead to cardiac insulin resistance in adult offspring.* Nutrition. 2008 Jul-Aug;24(7-8):727-32. Epub 2008 May 21.

242   Berg JM, Tymoczko JL, Stryer L. 2002. *Biochemistry, 5th Edition,* Retrieved from https://www.ncbi.nlm.nih.gov/books/NBK21190/.

243   Mozaffarian D, Pischon T, Hankinson SE, Rifai N, Joshipura K, Willett WC, Rimm EB. *Dietary intake of trans fatty acids and systemic inflammation in women.* Am J Clin Nutr. 2004 Apr;79(4):606-12.

244   Mozaffarian D, Rimm EB, King IB, Lawler RL, McDonald GB, Levy WC. *Trans fatty acids and systemic inflammation in heart failure.* Am J Clin Nutr. 2004 Dec;80(6):1521-5.

245   Qian JY, Leung A, Harding P, LaPointe MC. *PGE2 stimulates human brain natriuretic peptide expression via EP4 and p42/44 MAPK.* Am J Physiol Heart Circ Physiol. 2006 May;290(5):H1740-6. Epub 2006 Jan 20.

246   Nutrition Science News. http://www.newhope.com/nutritionsciencenews/ NSN_backs/Jul_99/dialogue.cfm Accessed 7/21/07.

247   Najib S, Sanchez-Margalet V. *Homocysteine thiolactone inhibits insulin signaling, and glutathione has a protective effect.* J Mol Endocrinol. 2001 Aug;27(1):85-91.

248   Jakubowski H. *Molecular basis of homocysteine toxicity in humans.* Cell Mol Life Sci. 2004 Feb;61(4):470-87.

249   Ibid.

250   Huang RF, Huang SM, Lin BS, Hung CY, Lu HT. *N-Acetylcysteine, vitamin C and vitamin E diminish homocysteine thiolactone-induced apoptosis in human promyeloid HL-60 cells.* J Nutr. 2002 Aug;132(8):2151-6.

251   Chwatko G, Jakubowski H. *Urinary excretion of homocysteine-thiolactone in humans.* Clin Chem. 2005 Feb;51(2):408-15. Epub 2004 Dec 2.

252   Nutrition Science News. http://www.newhope.com/nutritionsciencenews/ NSN_backs/Jul_99/dialogue.cfm Accessed 7/21/07.

253   Roblin X, Pofelski J, Zarski JP. *[Steatosis, chronic hepatitis virus C infection and homocysteine].* Gastroenterol Clin Biol. 2007 Apr;31(4):415-20.

254   Adinolfi LE, Ingrosso D, Cesaro G, Cimmino A, D'Antò M, Capasso R, Zappia V, Ruggiero G. *Hyperhomocysteinemia and the MTHFR C677T polymorphism promote steatosis and fibrosis in chronic hepatitis C patients.* Hepatology. 2005 May;41(5):995-1003.

255   The Free Dictionary. http://medicaldictionary.thefreedictionary.com/ hepatic+steatosis, Accessed 7/25/07

256   Roblin X, Pofelski J, Zarski JP. *[Steatosis, chronic hepatitis virus C infection and homocysteine].* Gastroenterol Clin Biol. 2007 Apr;31(4):415-20.

257   Osborne, TF. Sterol Regulatory Element-binding Proteins (SREBPs): Key Regulators of Nutritional Homeostasis and Insulin Action. J. Biol. Chem., Vol. 275, Issue 42, 32379-32382, October 20, 2000.

258   Namekata K, Enokido Y, Ishii I, Nagai Y, Harada T, Kimura H. *Abnormal lipid metabolism in cystathionine beta-synthase-deficient mice, an animal model for hyperhomocysteinemia.* J Biol Chem. 2004 Dec 17;279(51):52961-9. Epub 2004 Oct 4.

259   Nutrition Science News http://www.newhope.com/nutritionsciencenews/ NSN_backs/Jul_99/dialogue.cfm Accessed 7/22/07

260   Daemon, MA, van 't Veer, C, Denecker, G, Heemskerk, VH, Wolfs, TG, Clauss, M, Vandenbeele, P, Buurman, WA. *Inhibition of apoptosis induced by ischemia-reperfusion prevents inflammation.* J Clin Invest. 1999 Sep;104(5):541-9.

261   Touch Briefings. http://www.touchcardiology.com/files/article_pdfs/ ept031_t_Axis.pdf Accessed 7/22/07.

262   Ibid.

263   Brosnan JT, Jacobs RL, Stead LM, Brosnan ME. *Methylation demand: a key determinant of homocysteine metabolism.* Acta Biochim Pol. 2004;51(2):405-13.

264   Touch Briefings. http://www.touchcardiology.com/files/article_pdfs/ ept031_t_Axis.pdf Accessed 7/22/07.

265   McNulty H, Dowey le RC, Strain JJ, Dunne A, Ward M, Molloy AM, McAnena LB, Hughes JP, Hannon-Fletcher M, Scott JM. *Riboflavin lowers homocysteine in individuals homozygous for the MTHFR 677C->T polymorphism.* Circulation. 2006 Jan 3;113(1):74-80. Epub 2005 Dec 27.

266   Gropper SS, Smith JL, Groff JL, Advanced Nutrition and Human Metabolism, 4ᵗʰ Edition, Thomson Wadsworth, USA, pg. 284.

267   Ibid. pg. 442.

268   Das S, Snehlata, Das N, Srivastava LM. *Role of ascorbic acid on in vitro oxidation of low-density lipoprotein derived from hypercholesterolemic patients.* Clin Chim Acta. 2006 Oct;372(1-2):202-5. Epub 2006 May 15.

269   Turley SD, West CE, Horton BJ. *The role of ascorbic acid in the regulation of cholesterol metabolism and in the pathogenesis of artherosclerosis.* Atherosclerosis. 1976 Jul-Aug;24(1-2):1-18.

270   Rossi CS, Siliprandi N. *Effect of carnitine on serum HDL-cholesterol: report of two cases.* Johns Hopkins Med J. 1982 Feb;150(2):51-4.

271   Argani H, Rahbaninoubar M, Ghorbanihagjo A, Golmohammadi Z, Rashtchizadeh N. *Effect of L-carnitine on the serum lipoproteins and HDL-C subclasses in hemodialysis patients.* Nephron Clin Pract. 2005;101(4):c174-9. Epub 2005 Aug 9.

272   Combs, Gerald F Jr. The Vitamins: Fundamental Aspects in Nutrition and Health, 3ʳᵈ Edition, Elsevier, NY, 2008. pg. 153.

273 Gropper, SS, Smith, JL, Groff, JL, <u>Advanced Nutrition And Human Metabolism., 4th Edition</u>. Thomson/Wadsworth, USA, 2005, pg. 270.

274 Comb, GF, Jr, PhD, <u>The Vitamins: Fundamental Aspects in Nutrition and Health</u>, Third Edition, Elsevier, NY, 2008, pg. 358.

275 Comb, GF, Jr, PhD, <u>The Vitamins: Fundamental Aspects in Nutrition and Health</u>, Third Editions, Elsevier, NY, 2008, pg. 257.

276 Cahill L, Corey PN, El-Sohemy A. *Vitamin C deficiency in a population of young canadian adults.* Am J Epidemiol. 2009 Aug 15;170(4):464-71. Epub 2009 Jul 13.

277 Block G, Jensen CD, Dalvi TB, Norkus EP, Hudes M, Crawford PB, Holland N, Fung EB, Schumacher L, Harmatz P. *Vitamin C treatment reduces elevated C-reactive protein.* Free Radic Biol Med. 2009 Jan 1;46(1):70-7. Epub 2008 Oct 10.

278 Woodhouse PR, Meade TW, Khaw KT. *Plasminogen activator inhibitor-1, the acute phase response and vitamin C.* Atherosclerosis. 1997 Aug;133(1):71-6.

279 Swiatkowska M, Szemraj J, Cierniewski CS. *Induction of PAI-1 expression by tumor necrosis factor alpha in endothelial cells is mediated by its responsive element located in the 4G/5G site.* FEBS J. 2005 Nov;272(22):5821-31.

280 Makowsli, Gregory. <u>Advances in Clinical Chemistry</u>, *Volume 45*. Elsevier, Burlington, Ma, 2008, pg. 110.

281 Jone, David S, Editor in Chief. <u>The Textbook of Functional Medicine.</u> Gig Harbor, Wa. 2005, pg. 603.

282 Pivovarova, Olga, et al., *Modulation of insulin degrading enzyme activity and liver cell proliferation,* Cell Cycle. 2015 Jul 18; 14(14): 2293–2300.

283 Becker, Kenneth L, Bilezikian, John P, Bremner, William J, Hung, Wellington, Kahn, C Ronald. <u>Principles and Practice of Endocrinology and Metabolism. Third Edition.</u> Lippincott Williams & Wilkins, 2001 pg. 1274.

284 Becker, Kenneth L, Bilezikian, John P, Bremner, William J, Hung, Wellington, Kahn, C Ronald. <u>Principles and Practice of Endocrinology and Metabolism. Third Edition.</u> Lippincott Williams & Wilkins, 2001 pg. 1274.

285 Hernandez, Arturo PhD; St. Germain, Donald L. MD. *Thyroid hormone deiodinases: physiology and clinical disorders.* Current Opinion in Pediatrics: August 2003 - Volume 15 - Issue 4 - pp 416-420

286 Ibid.

287 Preedy, Victor R, Burrow, Gerard N, MD, Watson, Ronald. Comprehensive <u>Handbook of Iodine: Nutritional, Biochemical,</u>

Pathological and Therapeutic Aspects. Elsevier, Inc., Burlington, Ma, 2009, pg. 489.

[288] Wildman, Robert EC, Medeiros, Dennis M. Advanced Human Nutrition. CRC Press LLC, Boca Raton, Fla, 1999, pg. 185.

[289] Ibid.

[290] Packer, Lester, Fuchs Jurgen. Vitamin C in Health and Disease. Marcel Dekker, Inc, 1997, pg.39.

[291] Ibid.

Printed in the United States
By Bookmasters